D0778172

Intimacy After Cancer

A Woman's Guide

Intimacy After Cancer

A Woman's Guide

Dr. Sally Kydd and Dana Rowett

Big Think Media, Inc.

© 2006 Sally Kydd and Dana Rowett

All rights reserved. No part of this book may be reproduced in any form or by any means, electronic or mechanical, including photocopying, recording, or by any information or storage and retrieval system (including search engines), without the permission in writing from the publisher, except by a reviewer who may quote brief passages in a review.

Printed in the United States of America.

For information, visit us at Big Think Media, Inc., www.bigthinkmedia.com, or contact us at info@bigthinkmedia.com

Cover and book design by Katy Scott, www.katyscott.com

ISBN   0-9788108-0-5
         978-0-978810-80-1

Unless otherwise noted, names of individuals are fictional. Trade names of products are properties of their respective companies, and no consideration was either given or received in exchange. Products discussed in the book should not be construed as endorsement.

Although we strive to present only current and accurate information, readers should not consider it as professional advice, which can only be given by a healthcare provider. The views and opinions expressed in these pages are those of the authors. Although great care has been taken in compiling and checking the information given in this publication to ensure accuracy, the authors, Big Think Media, Inc., and its servants or agents shall not be responsible or liable in any way for the currency of the information or for any errors, omissions, or inaccuracies in this title, whether arising from negligence or otherwise howsoever or for any consequences arising therefrom.

The information you find in this book is not intended to be medical advice and does not specifically address any particular person's health care or other needs. It should not be used in place of a visit, call, consultation with, or advice of your own physician or other health care provider. If you have any health care-related questions or concerns, please call or see your health care provider promptly. You should never disregard medical advice or delay in seeking medical advice because of something you read here.

DEDICATIONS

To those who choose to live with
joy, intimacy and enthusiasm after cancer,
and in memory of those
who did not survive to make the choice.
Dr. Sally Kydd

To Bruce, who lived his life with gusto and passion,
and to the God who knows the answer
to the question "Why?"
Dana Rowett

Together, we would like to acknowledge
the many doctors and nurses
who dedicate their lives to fighting cancer
and its side effects.

We also acknowledge and dedicate this book
to all of the survivors and thrivers who continue to work hard
to reclaim a fulfilling life after cancer.
Dr. Sally Kydd
Dana Rowett

In Memory Of
Shashi S. Prasad
1937-2006

Loving family man and loyal friend

*An inspiration to all who knew him and
many who had only heard of him*

*He was instrumental in bringing together the
talented people who worked on this book*

*His charisma, commitment, and genuine fondness
and fairness for all is deeply missed*

Table of Contents

1. Kiss Me, I Had Cancer 1
   "How Did We Get Here, Toto?" 2
   What Happened To My Sex Life? 3
   What Are Common Intimacy Issues?. 5
   Do I Have Intimacy Issues? 6
   A Quiz To Help You Connect With The Issues 6
   Asking For Help 10
   And In Conclusion. 12

2. Am I Damaged Goods? 17
   Does This Make Me Look Fat? 19
   What Is Body Image? 22
   The Positive Police 23
   How Do You Like Me Now? 26
   Solutions To Body Image Problems 27
   Somebody Loves You 29
   A Little Helpful Information... 32

3. Self-Esteem: Me, Myself, and I 37
   Rosenberg Self-Esteem Scale 39
   Differentiation?. 41
   Solutions For Low Self-Esteem 42
   Cognitive Distortions 44
   Solutions To Cognitive Distortions 47
   Where I Come From.... 50

4. I'D RATHER READ A BOOK 55
   Motivation, Shmotivation! 57
   Use It Or Lose It? 59
   What If I'm (Not) In The Mood For Love? 61
   HEADLINE: Sex Goddess Reconnects The Sensory Neuron . . . 63
   Return To Your First Love... 64
   Loss Of Libido 66
   What Should I Expect After Treatment? 68
   Is It All In My Head? 69
   First, A Little Overview 71
   Common Side Effects Of Treatment 75
   Oh Goody...Early Menopause! 76

5. READING THE RIGHT BOOK 79
   What Can Be Done? 79
   The Fatigue Monster. 81
   Medications, Illness And Side Effects 83
   Hormone Therapy. 85
   Other Medications 87
   Your New Mantra: Lubricate, Lubricate, Lubricate! 88
   And Stretch...And Tone...Vaginal Aerobics? 91
   The Shrinking Violet...I Mean Vagina? 91
   Don't Forget To Bring The Humor. 93
   A Humming, Pleasant Road To Travel? 94
   What Are Other Options? 96
   Can I Use Bioidentical Hormones? 98
   Non-Herbal CAMs 99
   Developing Treatments. 102

6. MY HEART HURTS...STOLEN JOY 105
   Psychological Causes Of Lost Desire 106
   Depression Self-Test 107
   Other Psychological Challenges After Cancer 108
   Solutions To Common Psychological Intimacy Problems 110

Depression, Anger, Anxiety. 116

Solutions Continue. 120

Normal Aging Versus Cancer Symptoms 120

Sex And Infertility 123

Questions For Your Doctor. 124

7. BRING BACK THAT LOVING FEELING 129

Thursday Dinner Dates. 130

New Beginnings…Just Like Old Times 131

How Do I Set The Mood With An Ostomy Bag? 134

And Now…Let Us Begin Again! 135

"O" My!. 136

Four Counts To Lift Off. 137

I Did It All By Myself! 138

Annie, Get Your Vibrator… 140

Are You An "Inny" Or An "Outty"? 143

Up, Up, And Away!. 146

A Road Less Traveled? 150

8. HE SAID, SHE SAID 155

A Spouse Or A Louse. 156

Superman And Wonder Woman 157

I'll Love You Forever. 161

Communication Styles 162

Happy Talking Happy Talk? 164

Mistaking His Silence For Agreement 167

Begin The Beginning. 169

Look What We Done, Ma!. 171

9. SEX AND THE SINGLE WOMAN 175

Not By Choice… 177

By Choice… 178

Don't Cast Your Pearls Before Swine… 179

Now That You Know Better.… 184

Singles Need Sexual Support, Too! 184

Where To Find Dates After Treatment 185

Keep It Safe, Sister 186

We All Need Love 187

10. It's Not About Me When... 189

Thinking Like A Man...No Personalization! 190

External Personality Groups 191

TLC – Totally Ludicrous Comments? 191

Goodness Is About You! 198

11. For Husbands and Partners 199

Women Think Out Loud, And Men Take Action! 201

When Words Speak Louder Than Actions 203

Intimacy Versus Sex 205

Sex After Cancer: Just The Facts, Man 206

Playing Solitaire... 207

Bring Your Sense Of Humor... 208

Now, Do You Have A Minute To Talk? 209

12. Hidden Blessings 211

Resiliency, Anyone? 212

Blessed Stories 214

Flight For Life 215

A New Focus 215

Additional Blessings... 217

Post-Traumatic Growth 218

And They're Off...To The Races? 220

At Last...The Grand Finale! 221

Resource List 225

ACKNOWLEDGMENTS

Many health professionals and courageous survivors generously gave of their time and expertise to help us create this book. We thank you from the bottom of our hearts. Because of you, our readers have a tool on their journey to a better quality of life.

Dr. Sally Kydd: I extend my heartfelt thanks to the doctors and nurses who helped me get well when I was diagnosed with breast cancer: to Marsha Kooken, who has given generously of her expertise and was my personal guide through my breast cancer journey, for which I am forever grateful; to Dr. Eshwar Kumar, my oncologist, who has given a caring doctor's perspective and expertise; to Wendy Cyr, RN, a resource and guide as well as a source of encouragement to those of us who can help others on their cancer journey; to my intimacy and sexuality workshop co-presenter, Diana Leitch, R.N., who contributed to this book and to my personal growth, and who has encouraged me to talk, as she does, about the physical side of sexual issues; to Dr. Mary Beth Harman, a gynecologist and sex therapist, who contributed her expertise and kept us on track.

Giants in the field of sexuality after cancer and sex therapy are Dr. Leslie Schover and Dr. Sandra Leiblum, without whom this book would not be in existence. Dr. David Burns, a psychiatrist, who wrote about how to use cognitive therapy to handle anxiety and depressive disorders, provided the framework for the psychological approach to dealing with sexual issues after cancer. In addition, I thank Peggy Brick, Teri Henderson, Marianne Glasell, and others, some of who have chosen to remain anonymous, for their invaluable contributions in helping the ideas behind the book eventually emerge onto the printed page.

Finally, I want to acknowledge the contribution of the Canadian Breast Cancer Foundation and MindCare, New Brunswick, part of the Saint John Regional Hospital Foundation, for providing a grant for workshops on intimacy and sexuality after cancer. The material covered in these workshops acted as a framework for issues discussed in the book.

This book was not written in a vacuum. My co-author, Dana Rowett, has been a joy to work with and is gifted in taking challenging concepts, researching them thoroughly, and converting them to understandable written text. My husband, Barry, has always encouraged me to become all that I can be, and has been a wonderful, loving partner for forty years. My mother, Dinah Norman, who died of breast cancer in 2000, modeled caring and compassion to everyone with whom she came into contact. I hope I absorbed some of it from her. And, in conclusion, I want to thank my son, Angus, who has brought such joy and meaning to my life.

Dana Rowett: Thanks to all of the brave women who allowed me to ask them very personal, intimate, and sometimes embarrassing questions so we could write a book for women just like them. All my thanks to Becky Olson, Pam Bartholomew, Kathy LaTour, Linda Dackman, Susan Merrill, and Cindy Smith, who generously let me into their love lives and personal battles with cancer. I admire each of you greatly. In addition to the health professionals mentioned by Dr. Sally, thanks go to Subha Addy, M.S.W. and to Jackie Manthorne at the Canadian Breast Cancer Network. These women are warriors in the battle against cancer.

Thank you to my husband, Bob, and my sons Ben and Bobby for being patient and supporting me throughout this process, even when I turned their media room into my "war room." Thanks to my sister, Jennifer, who offered constructive criticism, and to my family and friends who never failed to encourage me. Last, but not least, I thank my co-author, Dr. Sally Kydd, whose direct, loving, compassionate, and generous spirit and intellect made this the most enjoyable work experience of my life. How lucky I am to know you! Now the world will know you too.

Together, we would like to thank the team that helped produce the book: Arushi Sinha, Ph.D., our incredible and amazing publisher; Katy Scott, our talented book designer; Cynarah Alcantara, our dedicated project manager; Dan Fernandez, our copy editor, and Richard Howdy, our medical illustrator, the two brave, professional, and talented men on our team.

We hope you enjoy the fruits of our combined labor.

DR. SALLY KYDD'S JOURNEY

I have always wanted to be a clinical psychologist as I have always been fascinated with what makes people "tick." I became interested in helping people deal with grief and loss following the death of our daughter over 20 years ago. I understood the pain of loss through death, and thought that I could give meaning to her short life by helping others through similar pain. Well, I have had some more "loss" experiences since then that have enabled me to arrive at a place where maybe I can help others to deal with issues following cancer. Let me explain.

My mother was diagnosed with breast cancer in 1989 and I understood, for the first time, what it felt like to be a family member of someone who had cancer. She was remarkably self-sufficient and well adjusted as she went through her radiation treatments. She coped as she always did, focusing on other people, never herself. Issues of sexuality were never discussed. Unfortunately, her cancer returned some years later, and she died in 2000.

In 2002, I was diagnosed with breast cancer, and I immediately realized how different it is when you are the one who has cancer. Although I had a wonderful medical team, issues of sexuality were almost never discussed. Only one doctor, my gifted, very special mastectomy surgeon, Dr. Robert Cowgill in Atlanta, talked about how my surgery would impact my sex life. I chose to have a double mastectomy and "free tram" reconstruction. Dr. Cowgill warned me that by undergoing this procedure, "you will never have any sexual pleasure from your breasts again." He gave me the opportunity to weigh my options in terms of how my treatment would impact my sex life and, for this, I am forever grateful.

I am co-authoring this book now because I had to find out for myself how to deal with the sexual issues that arose after my surgery, and as a result of taking medications to prevent any recurrence of the disease. I want to share what I have learned with the many women who have had cancer, and to offer you the hope that all aspects of your life, including your intimate life, can be as good, or better, after your illness than it was before.

After my surgery, I wasn't happy with my scarred body, I didn't think it looked nice, and it didn't "work" as well any longer. Emotionally, I felt traumatized and didn't understand what was happening. I realized that all my psychological training had not fully prepared me for what I was now facing. I was now coping with a different kind of loss, the loss of my body as I knew it, the loss of my sense of invulnerability, the loss of who I thought I was, and I was beginning to feel so very mortal. Not only was my body physically different; parts of my body, including my breasts, had no feeling at all – like, NO feeling. And, into all this mix, I questioned whether I was still desirable to my husband. Was I still a sexual being? How could I overcome the effects of tamoxifen, which caused my sex drive to disappear and my body to change in ways that made intercourse painful?

It has been a long journey, an interesting journey, taken with an understanding, wonderful partner, and learning from many giants in the field of sexuality after cancer. There is real hope for those of us who have had cancer, and want to continue to enjoy life to the fullest. Your intimate life can be immensely fulfilling, such that you become much more "alive" in every aspect of your existence after cancer than you were before. My hope is that you can benefit from what my co-author Dana Rowett and I have learned about how to overcome both the physical and psychological impact of cancer treatment on your intimate life .

One final, significant, challenge for me, in overcoming sexual issues after I had cancer, is that I am very private in terms of talking about my own sexuality. I know I am not alone in this. One advantage of my psychological training is that, when I don't know something, I know how to search for solutions. I have had to overcome my own reticence in talking about sex, and challenge my doctors to help me find solutions. If I can do it, you can too. If your doctors are shy or embarrassed (very likely), lacking in knowledge or unwilling (less likely) to help you overcome sexual issues related to your diagnosis, read this book, get educated, and get assertive. If they are unable to help, ask for referrals. Be your own champion, and get the answers you need to live the life you want.

DANA AND SALLY TOGETHER

Dana Rowett and I were introduced through our publisher and a wonderful writing journey began for the two of us. Dana's passion for empowering the average person with the knowledge needed to make the best health decisions combined with my passion to help others deal with grief and loss have made for a wonderful partnership. Dana lost a beloved brother to cancer and understands, as a support person, the stressors of endless doctors appointments, the side effects of chemotherapy and radiation, and the feeling of the bottom dropping out when the news worsens. Dana and I interviewed many experts in the field of cancer and sexual health and attempted to create a safe place where you could find the answers to your questions.

We hope you realize after reading this book that your concerns and current sexual issues are valid. They are not all in your head, and you are not alone. Many women have the same issues that you have after cancer treatment; it's just that we're not openly discussing them yet. We hope to change all of that.

The information you find in this book is not intended to be medical advice and does not specifically address any particular person's health care or other needs. It should not be used in place of a visit, call, consultation with, or advice of your own physician or other health care provider. If you have any health care-related questions or concerns, please call or see your health care provider promptly. You should never disregard medical advice or delay in seeking medical advice because of something you read here.

You should also know that, unless otherwise noted, all of the names in our book are fictitious. Names denoted with an asterisk (*) are imaginary and represent a composite of common concerns voiced by many women who responded to surveys and interview questions. Trade names of products are properties of their respective companies, and no consideration was either given or received in exchange for providing such information in this book. Product discussions in the book should not be construed as endorsements.

We want to emphasize the importance of safety when you are trying new ways to make love. Your immune system may be weakened from treatment, and safe, gentle lovemaking is key. Each of us is different and has a unique medical history. Talk with your doctor about your own personal health needs before trying any suggestions in this book.

Also, we have used the terms "partner," "lover," "husband," or "mate" throughout this book. We do not wish to be insensitive to women in same-sex relationships, but found it difficult to consistently use the words "he" and "she" throughout when discussing your partner. We also discovered through the course of writing this book that while same sex partners also experience issues arising from sexual, body image, and communication problems after cancer treatment, often, the two women in the relationship are more open to trying new ways of making love and communicating about sex (although this is not true across the board). However, both heterosexual and homosexual relationships are implied throughout the book.

Medical information is always changing as new information is discovered. We have attempted to provide you with the most current, up-to-date medical information that was available at the time of this printing. However, ask your doctor about the newest treatments that are available to you.

Because of all of the complicated medical terminology you've had to learn throughout your treatment, it was our intent to give you a book that you could read at your leisure…as if you were discussing these issues with trusted friends over a cup of tea. We hope you feel comforted and empowered after reading this book. We also hope you find the answers to your questions, or at least learn where to go for the answers. We wish you a safe, enjoyable journey back to a strong, healthy love life.

Dr. Sally Kydd and Dana Rowett
August 15, 2006

THE WORLD HEALTH ORGANIZATION
DEFINES HEALTH AS:

*Health is a state of complete physical, mental and social well-being
and not merely the absence of disease or infirmity.*

O N E

Kiss Me, I Had Cancer

Ruth* looked up from her hospital bed and smiled a big, beautiful smile. She was recovering from a complete hysterectomy to treat cervical cancer. Five years ago, Ruth had a double mastectomy for breast cancer. She was now in her 70s with no breasts and no uterus. But Ruth was thrilled to see her husband who was coming to take her home. She grinned again and whispered to me, "He still chases me around the house!"

Marsha Kooken, Oncology Nurse

e all need to feel the kind of closeness that comes from being held, kissed, hugged, and loved. Intimacy in a relationship improves the quality of our lives. But how can you return to a desire for intimacy after the trauma and treatment of cancer? Perhaps you have the desire but are afraid of how your partner will respond. Maybe you are single and wonder about dating. One thing is for certain: you are changed both inside and out. Your needs and desires might be different than they once were.

"HOW DID WE GET HERE, TOTO?"
ASKS DOROTHY AFTER A VICIOUS CYCLONE DROPS HER INTO THE LAND OF OZ.

First, the cancer diagnosis suddenly and cruelly invaded your life. Next, months of treatment probably left you fatigued, without hair, perhaps disfigured, and possibly with symptoms of sudden-onset (acute) menopause. Who feels sexy after this? If intimacy means taking off your clothes and using energy you just don't have, then forget it. Sitting down to read a good book might be the only intimacy you want. Still, don't be too quick to give up the intimate moments of your life. You can become a sexual person again, even if you're not entirely sure you want to awaken that part of your life.

Our society tells us that in order to be desired, we should be young, thin, urban women with big, heaving breasts walking around in expensive high-heeled shoes ready to slip into that perfect little negligee for hours of orgasmic sex. These expectations were unnatural before cancer. However, in truth, even our previous "normal" sexual relationship may be altered after cancer treatment. No one warned us there could be a time when we had to first remove a prosthetic breast, make sure an ostomy bag was properly sealed to prevent leaking urine, tuck away a drainage bulb, or apply a lubricant to our vagina before we slip into bed for that big romantic moment. The reality of our new sex life is not what we thought it would be. We must adjust our thinking. We may also need to adjust the way we find pleasure in our relationships, both physically and emotionally.

> ❖ *Intimacy is not just about sexual intercourse and multiple orgasms. Intimacy involves being valued as a human being by another human being.*

Intimacy is not just about sexual intercourse and multiple orgasms. Intimacy involves being valued as a human being by another human being.

As Becky Olson, cancer survivor and professional public speaker says, "Hugs are huge," especially as you move through the treatment stages of cancer and into recovery. Some of Becky's intimate moments with her husband came as little surprises. For instance, while Becky was having chemotherapy treatments, her husband was home cleaning the toilet because he knew she would be hugging it soon. Without her asking, Becky's husband made sure she had a sanitary place to wrap her arms and lay her head. He also stroked the back of her neck and whispered supportive words as she repeatedly vomited, and then he promptly cleaned up the mess when it was over. Now that's love. This kind of closeness helped Becky and her husband talk about her physical and emotional needs as she progressed through treatment and recovery.

WHAT HAPPENED TO MY SEX LIFE?

Some cancer treatments can trigger sudden-onset menopause. You may end up with hot flashes, fatigue, a lack of sexual desire, and symptoms such as a dry vagina that makes intercourse painful. Even if you don't have menopausal symptoms, cancer treatments such as chemotherapy and radiation can drain your energy and cause you to gain weight. Then of course, there are the surgeries to remove breasts, a uterus and ovaries, or to remove a diseased colon or intestine and attach an ostomy bag. What woman wants to have wild, passionate sex after these types of major physical and emotional changes?

Emotionally, your intimacy issues may depend upon the type of relationship you had before you were diagnosed with cancer. If you and your partner were good communicators before you developed cancer, you will probably continue to be during treatment and recovery. If you had an active sex life beforehand, you possibly will maintain the desire for sex throughout treatment and beyond, although it is also possible that your desires will change. If you struggled with communication or did not have an active sex life before cancer appeared, you and your partner may continue to have difficulty in these areas. Cancer can be a bonding experience for some couples as they share their fears and support each other; however, it can also add to existing problems and tear couples further apart. A crisis like cancer brings out both the best and worst in people.

Wendy Cyr, RN, a Case Manager at the Atlantic Health Science Corporation in New Brunswick, Canada tells a "best case" story about a woman who was hospitalized for advanced cancer:

> *The woman with cancer and her husband were quite attractive, so much so that hospital staff playfully referred to them as Mr. and Mrs. Gorgeous. The husband was unconditionally supportive and attentive to his wife during her treatment. When the wife became ill and was no longer comfortable having her husband in her hospital bed during his visits, Mr. Gorgeous asked the staff to place an extra bed beside his wife's. For an entire month, he lay next to her and simply held her hand, the only comfort he could provide without causing her pain. Intimacy was still important to this couple, even when she was too ill to do anything but hold hands. Mr. Gorgeous made sure his wife received the kind of intimacy she needed even at the end of her life. The hospital staff saw that he was gorgeous both inside and out.*

On the flip side, some partners are unable to provide all of the emotional or physical support a woman needs. Some relationships don't survive the stress of this crisis, although usually, these were not good relationships to begin with. Still, be careful about jumping to conclusions about the strength of your relationship. It's just possible your partner isn't as supportive as you'd like because he/she is not strong enough to watch you go through treatment. This weakness doesn't mean your relationship is doomed. It may mean that you and your partner will have to find other ways to feel connected through and after your battle with cancer. It also means that you will have to find support from another source. If your partner is unable to attend chemotherapy or other treatments, it's important to have another person with you. A good friend can hold your hand and make you laugh. Also if your partner won't discuss your concerns about sexual issues, then talk with a trusted friend who can give you courage while you seek the help you need. This is no time to be shy about asking for support.

WHAT ARE COMMON INTIMACY ISSUES?

The most common intimacy issues reported by women after cancer treatments include:

1. Losing the desire for sex
2. Worrying about the appearance of a new body and a partner's response to it
3. Experiencing pain during lovemaking

If you have one or all of these issues, you are not alone. A study by Dr. Patricia Ganz, MD, University of California – Los Angeles, Jonsson Comprehensive Cancer Center, and her colleagues, reports a high rate of symptoms such as joint pain, headaches, and hot flashes in women undergoing cancer treatment. Younger women tend to complain more often of sexual difficulties and intimacy issues after cancer treatment, although older women experience these problems too. The good news is that after cancer treatment, the women in the study eventually found the quality of their sexual functioning to be equal to or better than that of healthy women in their age group. Because women often do not seek professional care for sexual problems, the study's authors advise health professionals to encourage women to seek help with managing sexual symptoms. The sooner women seek help, the sooner they return to a healthy quality of sexual functioning.[1]

It is unfortunate, but not surprising that we as women often do not talk about these "embarrassing secrets" and are not regularly asked about our sexual health by our doctors. It is the painful secret we keep to ourselves, and it's a growing problem as more women are diagnosed with cancers.

Your sexual health is an incredibly important part of your whole well-being. It is essential that you feel free to discuss these issues openly with your partner, doctors, nurses, and other health professionals. These questions require satisfactory answers. Bottom line: Talk about your sexual issues with your partner, therapist, doctor, and nurse until you get the help you need. You don't have to live feeling disconnected, unloved, or without intimacy in your life.

DO I HAVE INTIMACY ISSUES?

If you have to ask the question, chances are that you have some intimacy or sexual issues in your life. Hopefully, you will feel validated and reassured by knowing that numerous women who have battled or are battling cancer have faced the same intimacy issues that you face. Unfortunately, many women do not ask the questions and, instead, choose to tune out this important part of their lives. The answers are out there. We hope to provide you with the answers to important questions in this book, but it can't stop here. Please follow through and do whatever it takes to improve the quality of your sexual life. It is crucial to seek appropriate help from your partner and your health professionals.

In Dr. Leslie Schover's book, <u>Sexuality and Fertility After Cancer</u>, she states:[2]

> *Cancer and sex are two words that do not seem to belong in the same sentence. We think of sexuality as a force for joy and new life, whereas cancer is a death force...Being able to enjoy sex is one important battle in winning the war against cancer.*

A QUIZ TO HELP YOU CONNECT WITH THE ISSUES

There are many mistaken beliefs about what happens to a woman's sex life after she has cancer. For instance, some women think intimacy in general is no longer a viable part of their lives. The following quiz may help connect you with your own intimacy issues and also give a better understanding of the truths and the myths of women's sexuality and intimacy issues after cancer.

SEXUALITY AFTER CANCER: TRUE/FALSE QUIZ

Take a guess and see what you know about common intimacy issues surrounding women just like you. Mark "T" or "F" before each sentence.

1. ___ Women's sexual problems after cancer are always due to reduced estrogen.

2. ___ The best measure of how your sex life will be after cancer is your sex life before cancer.

3. ___ During chemotherapy, it is recommended that couples refrain from having sex.

4. ___ The way a woman perceives her own body after cancer is pretty similar to how others perceive it.

5. ___ For a woman to be satisfied after sexual intercourse, it is important that she achieve orgasm.

6. ___ Effective communication is an important factor in satisfactory sexual functioning.

7. ___ Your oncologist is the best person to speak to about any sexual concerns you may have.

8. ___ A woman's most important sexual organ is located in her genital area.

9. ___ Medications taken to prevent recurrence of cancer, such as tamoxifen, are the most likely causes of sexual dysfunction in a survivor.

10. ___ Sexual self-stimulation or self-pleasuring after cancer should not be practiced.

11. ___ Physical exercise and a healthy diet can help a person's level of sexual desire increase.

12. ___ You should not tell a potential sexual partner that you have had cancer until you are in bed with him or her.

13. __ Different types of mental or physical sexual stimulation may increase sexual desire after cancer.

14. __ It is important to be spontaneous with your partner when choosing to have sexual intercourse.

15. __ Effective vaginal lubrication can allow women to enjoy pain-free sexual activity after cancer.

16. __ Couples are more likely to divorce once one partner has had cancer.

ANSWER KEY

1. FALSE.   Reduced estrogen levels account for some of the reduction in desire, but there are other factors such as religious beliefs, relationship problems, and psychological factors such as depression.[3]

2. TRUE. If your sex life was satisfying and enjoyable prior to your diagnosis, it is more likely to continue to be pleasurable afterwards.

3. FALSE. Sexual activity during chemotherapy is usually safe. Premenopausal women may become pregnant, so they should use contraceptives. If your immune system is severely depressed, it may be necessary to be more creative in expressing your sexual enjoyment of each other.[4]

4. FALSE. If you had cancer and subsequent scars or other bodily changes, you may be more critical of your own appearance than your partner. You might be worried that your partner will no longer be attracted to you.

5. FALSE. Research has shown that the top three items women associate with satisfying sex are feeling loved, feeling close to a partner before sex, and feeling emotionally close afterwards.[5]

6. TRUE.   According to Dr. Leslie Schover, a leading researcher in sexuality after cancer, communication with one's partner is a "crucial step in recovering a satisfying sex life after cancer treatment."[6]

7. FALSE. The first person you need to speak to about your sexual concerns is your partner. Your oncologist may be an excellent person to talk to about your sexuality if the sexual problem is directly related to your cancer treatment, but he or she is not the only person. A gynecologist may help you overcome painful intercourse. A primary care doctor may also be helpful. However, these medical professionals may NOT be comfortable talking about your sexuality, in which case you may request a referral to a mental health professional with special training in sex therapy.

> *The first person you need to speak to about your sexual concerns is your partner.*

8. FALSE. A woman's MOST important sexual organ is her brain.

9. FALSE. Although taking tamoxifen can cause changes to the vaginal area, the more likely cause of sexual problems after cancer is chemotherapy treatment.[7]

10. FALSE. Sexual self-stimulation can help you reconnect with your own sexuality, if it is acceptable with your own and your religion's belief system. It can enable you to regain sexual interest when you may be too tired for sexual intercourse with a partner. Self-stimulation can also enable you to learn more about what is pleasurable, which you can later share with your partner.

11. TRUE. Physical exercise enables you to feel good about the fact that your body is still functioning. It has been shown to be effective in treating depression. Proper diet and exercise can also enhance sexual pleasure.[8]

12. FALSE. While there is no "right" time to tell a new sexual partner about your history of cancer, or about a lumpectomy, mastectomy, or other surgery, you might want to have this discussion before the two of you become sexually intimate.

13. TRUE. In order to reignite your physical sexual desire, it is important to stimulate your mind and increase your sexual imagination.

14. FALSE. You may have to plan a little bit for sex at first. Spontaneous lovemaking may have to be sacrificed for a short time during and after treatment for cancer so that sex can be enjoyable and pain-free.

15. TRUE. Lubrication can be effective in minimizing or eliminating painful sex after cancer.

16. FALSE. A number of surveys show that divorce rates don't increase after one partner has cancer.[9]

ASKING FOR HELP

Asking the right care provider the right questions can be tricky. If you think you have issues with intimacy or sexual functioning, help is certainly available. The problem can be in knowing where to turn for the answers. Many of the doctors who treat cancer are focused solely on saving lives; some may not take the time or know how to talk to their patients about sexual issues. However, this does not mean your doctors won't know where to send you for help. If you have concerns about sexual function or the quality of your intimate relationship, don't hesitate to talk with your health care professionals.

Recently, 300 women with cancer were asked the following questions: Who helped you with intimacy issues, and what kinds of helpful information were you given? Of the women who responded, many said they had not asked for help. Of those who did ask, half were disappointed with the information provided by their health professionals. These women first spoke to a family member or friend and then to their family doctor about their intimacy issues after cancer treatment; a few women talked with their oncologists. Most preferred to get this information from a book, pamphlet or Web site first, and then from their doctor or nurse, a support group, or from a lecture or conversation with a fellow survivor. In this book, we hope to present you with answers to questions you are afraid to ask. We'll also identify additional resources to help you get the conversation started with your health professional.

WHICH HEALTH PROFESSIONAL DO I TURN TO FOR HELP?

Since being diagnosed with cancer, you've probably met with several different health care professionals. The types of providers on your medical team depend upon what kind of cancer you have, how it is treated, and where you live. For instance, if you live in a larger city, you might have access to more types of care providers than if you live in a more rural, less populated area. Your medical team may consist of one or more of the following:

Medical Oncologist: The doctor who diagnoses the type and extent of cancer and treats it, usually with chemotherapy.

Radiation Oncologist: The doctor who treats cancer with radiation therapy.

Surgeon: The doctor who removes the cancer with appropriate surgery.

Oncology Case Manager: Usually a Registered Nurse (RN) with special training and education in caring for people with cancer. This person organizes your medical appointments, explains test results, and provides you with community resources.

Oncology Nurse: An RN with special training or certification in treating cancer who works with your doctor, hospital, or cancer care center.

Gynecologist: The doctor who often finds female cancers first and who may continue to provide you with care for common side effects of cancer treatments, such as vaginal wall thinning or dry vagina.

Primary Care Provider: This is usually your family doctor who may refer you to specialists but still monitor your care.

During active treatment, typically you'll see a medical or radiation oncologist more frequently than other providers. The oncologist may be able and willing to answer questions about sexuality, although the advice might be limited to how it relates to your cancer treatment (such as when is it safe to become sexually active during chemotherapy). Your gynecologist or primary care doctor might treat symptoms associated with treatment, such as painful intercourse, and may be the person you feel most comfortable with when discussing sexual concerns.

Please be aware, though, that some care providers may not be comfortable talking about your sexuality. Some women have been brave enough to ask their doctor only to be told "not to worry about sex right now." This is not an acceptable answer.

When talking to your doctor or other health professionals, you may want to ask a general question, such as, "I'm having sexual difficulties or concerns about intimacy; are you the person to talk with about this matter or can you refer me to the right person?" Your case manager or oncology nurse may also be a good resource for helping you find the right person to talk to about physical and emotional sexuality issues. Increasingly, there are many professional counselors, such as psychiatrists, psychologists, or licensed counselors or social workers, whose practice focuses on helping people with sexual or intimacy issues related to health problems.

AND IN CONCLUSION...

Especially as women, our brain is the biggest sex organ we have. It's not always about fulfilling a physical need, although that is part of it. It is about feeling whole, loved, and connected to our lover. Sexual intercourse does not always bring about this connection for women. You may not want to be touched at all, especially when going through cancer treatment. Intimacy is so much more than intercourse. Having your partner in the room with you, just sitting by your side, can be intimate and comforting. When you do feel like becoming

A woman's most important sexual organ is her brain.

sexual, you may not want to have intercourse. Touching, cuddling, holding hands, kissing, stroking, or just sitting together may be enough intimacy to connect you and your partner.

When cancer is first diagnosed, you are in survival mode and focused on doing whatever it takes to beat cancer. Attending doctors' appointments, deciding on treatment options, and successfully battling cancer are your primary goals. Sex likely falls to the bottom of your "to do" list. However, this does not mean you do not need intimacy in your relationship. Hugs, handholding, and quiet time with your partner are important. At this stage, your partner usually needs this type of intimacy too. If you are single, it is important that family members or friends provide you with hugs and other supportive touching. Cancer is scary, and you need the lifeline connection and energy that flows from unconditional love and support.

As you move through the stages of treatment, you may find that your need for intimacy changes. It can hurt to be touched. You may want to be left alone. Or you may find that you need reassurance and closeness from someone you love. Lying together with your partner, with clothes on or off, can be comforting and soothing. Holding hands while you talk about what's ahead or while you are reflective and quiet can build strength in your relationship.

It's important to remember that sometimes the people who love you can identify what you need and respond to your needs, but more often, you'll have to tell them what you are feeling and what you need from them. This is especially true for partners who become our caregivers and who often take over the bulk of responsibilities while we are fighting cancer. The combination of fear and lack of communication is a relationship breaker, but it's one that we can recover from if we communicate with our partner about our fears.

It's also important to distinguish the sexual side effects caused by cancer treatment from those that are a normal part of aging or are related to other stressors in your life (discussed more fully in Chapter Six). Ask yourself these questions: Were you sexually active prior to cancer? How did you and your partner express intimacy and love before you were diagnosed? Be careful not to blame cancer as the single cause of a limited sexual life, especially if it existed before cancer. Many healthy women are also not interested in sex, and the conflict about sex has been around for centuries. The following "urban legend"—a fabricated story, but humorous nonetheless—illustrates this common, ongoing struggle:

> *Many years ago, an astronaut took his first step on the moon. He echoed Neil Armstrong's famous words, "That's one small step for man, one giant leap for mankind." His next words were, "Good luck, Mr. Gorsky." Over the years, many people asked the astronaut what he meant, but he just smiled.*
>
> *Years later, a reporter insisted on knowing the meaning of the comment long ago uttered about Mr. Gorsky. Since Mr. Gorsky had died many years before, the astronaut succumbed to the persistent reporter. "You see, when I was a young boy playing baseball, I ran to catch a soaring ball under my neighbor's bedroom window. When I leaned down to pick up the ball, I heard Mrs. Gorsky shouting, 'Sex! You want sex?! You'll get sex when the kid next door walks on the moon!'"*

If this sounds too familiar, don't despair. Your health crisis can actually improve your sex life. Because women usually need to feel emotionally connected to a lover, cancer may prompt you to open up more about your needs, fears, desires, and hopes with your partner. Better communication can indeed lead to a more intimate relationship all around. And you won't have to wait until the kid next door lands on the moon!

FACT OR FICTION?

"Terminally ill people are not interested in sex."

FICTION! Even at the end of our lives, sex and intimacy are very important. We need to feel close or connected to another human being, especially someone we love.

---

[1] Ganz PA, Rowland, JH, et al. (1998). Life After Breast Cancer: Understanding Women's Health-Related Quality of Life and Sexual Functioning. Journal of Clinical Oncology, 16(2): 501-514.

[2] Schover LR (1997). Sexuality and Fertility After Cancer, p. xi. New York: John Wiley & Sons, Inc. Reprinted with permission of John Wiley & Sons, Inc.

[3] S. Leiblum (2002). The Role of the Sex Therapist in Female Sexual Dysfunction. New York University School of Medicine Conference. December 2002.

[4] Schover LR (1997). Sexuality and Fertility After Cancer, p. 52. New York: John Wiley & Sons, Inc. Reprinted with permission of John Wiley & Sons, Inc.

[5] Ellison CR (2000). Sexualities: Generations of Women Share Intimate Secrets of Sexual Self-Acceptance. Oakland, CA: New Harbinger Publication.

[6] Schover LR (1997). Sexuality and Fertility After Cancer, p. 30. New York: John Wiley & Sons, Inc. Reprinted with permission of John Wiley & Sons, Inc.

[7] American Cancer Society, Schover L (2004). Sexuality after Cancer for the Woman who Has Cancer and Her Partner. American Cancer Society.

[8] Hall K (2004). Reclaiming Your Sexual Self. Hoboken, NJ: John Wiley & Sons, Inc.

[9] Schover LR (1997). Sexuality and Fertility After Cancer, p. 8. New York: John Wiley & Sons, Inc. Reprinted with permission of John Wiley & Sons, Inc.

Two

Am I Damaged Goods?

*How do I get anyone to believe that I am desirable enough to
want me now? How do I make myself believe it?*
                                    Gina*, 44, breast cancer survivor

*V*iewing yourself as damaged goods after cancer treatment is
common. You may wonder if you are still a desirable woman.
You may ask yourself, "Do I still feel feminine without breasts or
reproductive organs?" Some changes that result from cancer treatment are
not so obvious; however, these changes still may impact the way you see
yourself.

Your attractiveness and sexuality are much more than having two
breasts, reproductive organs, or a perfect face and body. In a world where
the ideal woman's "perfect" though unrealistic physical appearance is
plastered over every advertisement, even women without cancer struggle
with body image. Combine this unrealistic image with a body altered by
cancer, and you can see why many cancer survivors have a difficult time
with self-assessment. To what, or with whom, do you compare yourself
now, after cancer? Is it the magazine photo of the 6-foot model with the

seemingly perfect body and teeth and long blond hair, who is lying on a beach with ocean waves spraying lightly over her perfect little breasts? We think not. In fact, maybe you should throw that magazine out. In reality, the photo of that woman is airbrushed to remove every stitch of cellulite, every wrinkle and spot. Her white teeth are dental caps, her hair is dyed and full of hair extensions, her perfect breasts are implants, and you can bet she has beach sand up her bottom. Free yourself from the bondage of unrealistic perfection; that image is not genuine beauty. It's not real…none of it.

Our bodies come in all shapes and sizes. As real women, we might have large hips, thighs, bellies, wrinkles, and sometimes flabby arms. We have beautiful smiles, unique swings in our walks, thoughts, ideas, and the ability to love unconditionally. We can turn that unconditional, compassionate love inward. We can love ourselves without measure, just the way we are.

You may have seen these "keyboard breasts" circulating on the Internet or in e-mails. We thought they were great examples of our wonderfully different bodies!

A CUPS o o	PUSH-UP BRA BREASTS (oYo)	D CUPS { O }{ O }
BIG NIPPLE BREASTS (@)(@)	PERKY BREASTS (*)(*)	LOPSIDED BREASTS (o)(O)
AGAINST THE SHOWER DOOR BREASTS ( )( )	PERFECT BREASTS (o)(o)	FAKE SILICONE BREASTS (+)(+)
COLD BREASTS (^)(^)	PIERCED BREASTS (Q)(O)	ANDROID BREASTS lol lol
	HANGING TASSELS BREASTS (p)(p)	

The relationship you have with yourself is the most important of all. Dorothy Rowe, an Australian psychologist, said in 1995 that the key to escaping depression is to simply become your own best friend. Yet we are often extremely self-critical. You can't expect to improve intimacy with your partner until you learn to love and accept the new you.

"How," you ask, "do I get past feeling like damaged goods?" By taking one step at a time. There are many issues after cancer or while living with cancer that affect your self-esteem. Most involve longing for a return to life as it was before cancer. In his book, <u>Breast Cancer Husband</u>, Marc Silver calls this preferring the "old normal" to the "new normal." [1] Your life has shifted. The bottom line is that it is impossible to return to your old normal. Something significant has happened, and your life will never be the same. However, this doesn't mean life, or your new normal, can't be better than it was before cancer. Much of it will be up to you. We can't always control what happens to us, but we can control how we respond to it.

This statement may be a little simplistic, especially after a life-altering diagnosis. Yet there is truth in it. Sometimes we must make a conscious decision to move forward, to change a negative attitude, or to get through legitimate grief by doing normal things until they feel normal again. All of this takes time, so be gentle to yourself on this journey.

DOES THIS MAKE ME LOOK FAT?

Before cancer, your concerns about body image probably focused on weight, or maybe what you saw as an unattractive feature, such as your nose or height. After all, ours is a culture obsessed with the female body image and impossible ideas of perfection. But what is your gauge for beauty now, after cancer? Let's "get real."

Here are a few facts:

- At any one time, more than half of the women in the United States are dieting.
- 40 years ago, the average woman was 12 pounds heavier than the top models; now she is nearly 30 pounds heavier (because models are thinner).

- Most supermodels are 5 ft. 10 in. and weigh 115 pounds.
- Women who are naturally tall and thin are also small breasted, so most models likely have had breast implants.
- The Playboy centerfold is now 25 pounds thinner than in 1986, and weighs 18% less than her ideal weight.
- The average woman sees about 400 to 600 advertisements every day that feature thin models pushing beauty products or clothing, making us believe this is the ideal image we should strive to attain.

Do you know the size of the average, normal-sized American woman? Most people think she is an 8, but a normal-sized American woman is a size 12. Marilyn Monroe, an American icon and a sex symbol since the 1950s, was a size 14! Mae West, sex goddess of the 1930s, was a size 14 (and sometimes a size 16). Today, however, thinness equals beauty, especially for women.

The truth is:

- Fashion models weigh 23% less than the average female (we're not talking an overweight female but an *average-sized* female).[2]
- Only 7% of young women ages 18 to 34 will ever be as slim as a runway model.
- Only 1% of women will ever be as thin as a supermodel.[3]

This is one area in today's culture where it might have been better to be a man. Why would anyone want to be this thin? If we can believe the reports, many models eat very little; they must induce vomiting, chain smoke, or take recreational drugs to stay this thin. It's not natural. Yet 69% of young girls surveyed said models had the perfect bodies.[4] Do you see the problem? Unrealistic body image leads to disappointment, frustration, feelings of failure, and self-loathing. When did we become so obsessed with unattainably skinny bodies? We need to stop thinking "waif-thin" and start thinking healthy – *especially* after cancer!

You were born with certain genetics that dictated your basic shape and looks. Tall, short, apple-shaped, pear-shaped, skinny, curvy; you can't change genetics, although we women sure do try. Anti-wrinkle creams, the newest fad diet, weight-loss equipment, or expensive make-up to make our noses look petite. We glom onto the newest fashion trends guaranteed to make us look thinner. It's exhausting being a woman in pursuit of advertising's view of physical perfection! We need to stop the madness and get real.

WOMEN   **MEN**

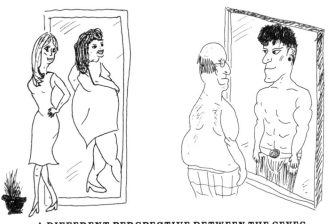

A DIFFERENT PERSPECTIVE BETWEEN THE SEXES

Nutrition, exercise, and feeling good about yourself are important, especially after cancer. If your body is altered since treatment, try to decide whether or not your new body image is affecting your self-esteem. Do you feel preoccupied with how you look since cancer? Medications, such as tamoxifen, can cause weight gain. Chemotherapy can leave you swollen, puffy, and possibly heavier than you once were. Maybe you have scars or missing body parts, or your body requires medical assistance, such as an ostomy bag. You may no longer be able to conceive. It's normal to resent your body and feel it betrayed you by developing cancer in the first place. You may not feel attractive or appealing. You might wonder if you'll ever accept the new you and if your partner will ever find you sexy after these changes. We won't keep you in suspense. The answer is a resounding, "YES!"

> *It's normal to resent your body and feel it betrayed you by developing cancer in the first place.*

WHAT IS BODY IMAGE?
Perfectionism + Reality = Self-Loathing

Body image is the mental picture you have about your body, and the way you treat yourself based on that image. We are usually our own worst critic. We take that unflattering image of ourselves and transfer it to the way we feel about ourselves generally as a person. Most of us fail the perfect body test. Of course, we easily excuse others with flawed bodies, but we are harsh about our own imperfections. That's the double standard we experience as women.

In her book, Love Your Looks, Carolynn Hillman writes that if a woman loves herself and treats herself with value, she is then able to love her own appearance. In our society, it's kind of the cart before the horse…liking yourself first, then liking the way you look. Carolynn says we shouldn't value ourselves only *after* we are satisfied with our looks. We should love the way we look *because we first value ourselves.* Love who you are, and sooner or later, you'll approve of your appearance – scars and all.

The problem is, many of us aren't that happy with how we look, and some of us don't like the person inside either. Much of our unhappiness with our appearance involves weight. This is true whether or not we've had cancer, although disfigurement after cancer may only make self-depreciation worse. Then again, cancer can also jolt us into reprioritizing our values, including reemphasizing the value of life, no matter what our appearance.

Feeling bad about your appearance filters into the bedroom. We don't want our imperfections seen, and therefore pull back both physically and emotionally from our lover. Does your negative body image affect your intimate relationship? To understand how you feel about your body now, after cancer, you have to understand your thought processes that affected your body image *before* your diagnosis.

Ask yourself, "Have I ever disliked my body? How do I feel about my body now? Do I dislike it more since cancer?" Most of us have at least one thing we would like to change about our looks. Does the way you feel about your appearance influence the way you feel about yourself on the inside? Do you have a negative view of your body that interferes with romance and intimacy? If the answers are yes, once again, you are not alone. Body image issues span across many cultures and affect many women.

In the past decade, women have disclosed that appearance was the number one reason for poor self-esteem. If a woman thought she was attractive, her self-esteem was high. The results haven't changed over time. More recently, Woman's Day magazine and America Online surveyed their readers about weight and appearance.[5] Thirty-five thousand people took this online survey! Of the women who responded, more than half thought they would feel more attractive if they lost weight. On the other hand, 68% of the men said they "loved how my partner looks." Remember, the average American woman is a size 12 and wants to lose weight. Yet 68% of men already loved how their wives and girlfriends looked AS THEY ARE RIGHT NOW!!!

In her documentary "Slim Hopes," Jean Kilbourne says that 75% of "normal" weight women think they are overweight, and 90% overestimate their body size.[6] Women compare themselves to other women, especially the unattainable thin model body types we mentioned earlier. Are you doing this, even subconsciously? Did you know that reading women's magazines will likely make you feel worse about your appearance?[7]

THE POSITIVE POLICE

Since cancer, your issue may not be weight so much as a missing breast or prominent scar. This new look will take some adjustment. And frankly, you don't have to feel happy about it while you are adjusting. You had cancer, the treatment left you disfigured and changed, and it stinks.

When asked or really told, "You must be so happy that your treatment is over," I always answer, "Yes, everything is GREAT!" I am so tired of everything always having to be "Sunshine and Gumdrops" and feeling guilty if I feel afraid, depressed, and fat. Now that I am trying to resume life as normal, I feel worse emotionally than at any time throughout treatment. Every day when I look in the mirror and see this curly hair and extra weight, I am reminded that cancer was in my body. I think I need the name of a good counselor.

Catherine McKinney, 41
Five months after surgery, radiation, and chemotherapy

When you add the "Swiss cheese" appearance after a lumpectomy or an unpleasant ostomy bag hanging from your side to an already narrow view of beauty, it's not a surprise that feeling attractive is a challenge. A lumpectomy can cause uneven breasts that appear different or look less appealing. Cancer surgeries sometimes remove sensation from the body. Your breasts may become numb or feel different. While reconstruction can recreate breasts where you once had scars, it's not a perfect solution. For example, a "free tram" breast reconstructive surgery uses your own stomach tissues to recreate your breasts. However, you'll loose sensation in your breast and stomach areas, and it may be challenging for you to feel that you "own" these parts of your body after surgery. In a society dominated by flawless examples of female beauty, a woman's self-confidence must be strong enough to sustain her self-esteem after her body is made less than perfect by cancer treatment.

There is so much written today about having a positive attitude that I try to keep it a secret if I have any negative thoughts.

Pauline*, 52
One year after a double mastectomy and reconstruction

Sometimes a positive attitude is just not doable. We may grow weary of people telling us to "be positive" after cancer. Hearing this little sentence repeatedly can transform even the most cheerful woman into an angry, irritated person. We all know that a "fighting spirit" is important. Dr. Matthew Cordova wrote about emotional suppression and a fighting spirit in cancer support groups.[8] He said that many cancer patients find it difficult to cope with intense feelings of fear, anxiety, sadness, and anger while at the same time being strongly encouraged by family, friends, and healthcare professionals to "stay positive" and "look on the bright side."

As a survivor and clinical psychologist, this book's co-author, Dr. Sally Kydd, has also been irritated by thoughtless comments. She believes it is important to maintain a sense of hope and optimism, but also to acknowledge both the positive and negative feelings about diagnosis and treatment.

> *It is important to maintain a sense of hope and optimism, but also to acknowledge both the positive and negative feelings about diagnosis and treatment.*

According to Dr. Cordova, it's not uncommon for you to become upset when someone tries to suppress or control your negative feelings. He says a fighting spirit refers to "facing difficult situations directly while at the same time maintaining hope." He suggests we accept strong negative emotions that come with a cancer diagnosis, but also change the threat so it is less overwhelming and easier to handle…and to our knowledge, this is quite different from "be positive!"

One way to change the threat is to learn how to process the realization and grief over the fact that your body is different. It is important not to "catastrophize" your situation. Very few situations are totally without hope. With ongoing cancer research, the prognosis for living a long life after a cancer diagnosis improves daily. You don't have to worry that every twinge you feel is terminal! You can learn to face the ups and downs with a sense of hope, while not feeling guilty when you have a "down" day.

While we know you can work through your loss, grief, and the adjustment of accepting your new body, we also understand that not every day will be a good day. If you feel lousy, it's important to find a safe place to express it, to a trusted doctor, counselor, friend, a cancer support group, or in a journal. "Stuffing" feelings of anxiety and sadness so everyone else sees you as "positive" is a sure way to end up with depression or other problems down the road.

As you move through this stage of your recovery, try to remember that you are more than a body part. Believe it or not, you can overcome apprehension about the new you since cancer. You might have to return repeatedly to the good advice of: Love yourself first, and then you can love your appearance.

HOW DO YOU LIKE ME NOW?
You, Your Partner, And Your Appearance

You, yourself, as much as anybody in the entire universe, deserve your love and affection.

Buddha

What do you and your mate find sexy? Did you know that most men like a sensual, voluptuous body? That means "provocative and sexually alluring, especially through shapeliness or fullness." Since some cancer medications, like tamoxifen, cause weight gain, you might be worrying about weight gain with treatment. But did you know that the Woman's Day/AOL survey showed that less than a quarter of men said a "svelte and trim body" was sexy? Has cancer treatment made you fuller and, therefore, more sexy? That is one way to look at it.

What about missing breasts? Where does voluptuous come into play with a flat, scarred chest? We want to be clear: Being voluptuous is not always about having big breasts. It's about the whole of you, your sensuality and a curvy body, which includes your bottom, thighs, and stomach. While you are focusing on what you don't have, your partner is focusing on the sensual parts you do have.

> *How you feel about your body impacts your willingness and ability to enjoy intimacy with your partner.*

Women tend to like their bodies less as they age. Generally, men don't go out of their way to be critical of us, especially during sex. You might be concerned about your stomach sagging when you are positioned on top during lovemaking, but your partner is *not* thinking about your stomach.

As women, we tend to "project" our own insecurities about our bodies onto our partner, believing he is thinking what we are thinking. For example, "her bottom is huge" or "she has no breasts, and I'm no longer turned on." Projection is a defense mechanism we use to protect ourselves emotionally from the anticipated rejection. The problem is, since a man is turned on by visual stimuli, he is focusing on what he finds beautiful about you, not what is missing. In fact, men are really turned off by women who fret about their bodies during sex.

While we can assure you that you are probably your own worst critic about body image, we also know it is important to feel comfortable with your body. How you feel about your body impacts your willingness and ability to enjoy intimacy with your partner.

> *It is hard to abandon yourself to the joys of sex if you're preoccupied with how your breasts are sagging, the flab on your body, the wrinkles on your face, or your stretch marks.*
> Carolynn Hillman
> in *Love Your Looks*

The fact is we use our bodies to become intimate or sexual with another person. If you feel bad about the way you look, you probably won't pursue sex or intimacy as easily in your relationship. The solution is to develop a kinder, more realistic appraisal of your body, and lose the negative image. When you succeed, you'll be able to relax and enjoy your partner sexually.

SOLUTIONS TO BODY IMAGE PROBLEMS
BECOMING A RADIANT WOMAN

Now that I've had radiation, I'm a radiant woman!
Lee*, 66

What made you feel attractive before cancer? Was it a physical attribute, such as your smile, eyes, breasts, or feet? Did you feel attractive because you had a certain talent, such as singing or painting? When did you feel flirtatious or aroused before your diagnosis? Go back to your first love. Go back to what made you feel warm down to your toes. If your breasts were your pride and joy but are now gone, you can find a new appeal. Find a new beautiful part of yourself previously left unexplored. Spend time looking at your body from head to toe. What do you find sexy about yourself now? If you discover a beautiful smile, then buy new shades of lipstick. Do you have lovely feet? Then have a pedicure or buy a new pair of shoes or both! Whatever it is about your body that you feel good about, emphasize it. Make a list of all the wonderful things about yourself, whether or not they reflect physical attributes. If you find this hard to do, try to imagine what you would say to someone else who looks just like you. Start feeling good about the radiant woman that you are. Love your inside self first, and then you can love your outside self.

We, as women, need to stop using **the double standard**, which is being kinder about other people's flaws than we are about our own. For instance, you may say another woman's breast reconstruction is beautiful, but say your own looks terrible. Look at yourself as kindly and gently as you look at others. Carolynn Hillman tells us to turn our inner *critic* into our inner *caretaker*. You must learn to **CARESS** yourself.

- Show **C**ompassion for whatever you are feeling about your looks and yourself
- Non-judgmentally **A**ccept you and your appearance
- **R**espect you for how you look and who you are
- **E**ncourage you to take steps and risks to achieve the things you want just as you look now
- **S**upport you by believing in you and reassuring you that how you look is just fine, and
- **S**troke you by praising your looks and giving you credit for trying.

If weight is or was your first body image issue, remember that in most cultures, bigger is better. Just because you live in a culture that prizes thinness doesn't mean it is correct. You are who you are. Your desire to be thin most likely does not match with your partner's desire of you either. However, if your partner is disapproving about your weight gain, give yourself permission to ignore those comments. You have to determine how you feel about yourself on your own, without interference or another critical voice.

SOMEBODY LOVES YOU
RESOURCES, RESOURCES, RESOURCES

If your body image issues since cancer treatment surround the loss of a body part, such as your breast(s), help is available. The American Cancer Society has a wonderful program called Reach to Recovery to help you improve your body image after cancer treatment, especially after losing a breast or breasts. Trained volunteers who are also cancer survivors assist you in adjusting to your altered body. These women have been where you are now. They offer you genuine support, wisdom, and hope for your future. Reach to Recovery volunteers can talk with you about breast prostheses and how to locate these items in your area (so can your doctor, if you prefer). Prostheses are sold in surgical supply stores, hospitals, and sometimes in the lingerie department of your favorite clothing store. The volunteers will teach you to dress to look your best after breast(s) removal, loss of hair, and other changes to your body since cancer treatment. We hope you will walk away from their loving guidance feeling like a sexy, strong woman. For more information, go online at: www.cancer.org and type in "Reach to Recovery" in the search box.

In addition, your local hospital or cancer treatment center should have similar resources to help you feel better about your new appearance after treatment. Be sure to check with your oncologist's office if your body image is suffering. Help is out there. If you are missing breast(s), special bras and breast prostheses might make you feel more comfortable in your clothing.

"That's a great help for when I'm dressed, but what about when I'm naked, especially in front of my partner?" you might ask. Your inhibition is perfectly understandable. However, it's only natural to first become more at ease with your body before you will become comfortable sharing it with your partner. Have you been able to look at your scar(s)? Until you are able to face them, you will probably try to hide them; and that's okay too, at least for a while. This is a painful step for many women. Even after you've viewed the scars, you may not be ready to share this part of your body with your partner. It turns out you don't have to, especially not one second before you are ready. However, you might be surprised by your husband or partner's response to the new you.

> *One of the most treasured moments of my life will always be the first time my husband kissed the scar where my breast used to be. I cried, but remember trying to hide the emotion from him, assuming he wouldn't understand. But then I recall crying, or stifling tears, frequently during those first few intimate moments, so thrilled was I to be alive and to be feeling so loved and accepted. Passion was secondary in those early months to the pockets of grief that tended to surface during lovemaking.*
> *Kathy LaTour, breast cancer survivor and author of The Breast Cancer Companion*

Until you are ready to be naked in front of your partner, you can wear special lingerie that covers lumpectomy and mastectomy scars and also abdominal scars or ostomy bags. You can feel sexy and beautiful without feeling self-conscious. You may keep it on during lovemaking or even cuddling. The lingerie comes in all sorts of styles, from silky pastels to textured wild animal prints. You can purchase this lingerie from the comfort of your own home if you like from Web sites such as www.nottiwear. com. Lingerie is also available with bilateral soft pockets to hold breast prostheses on such Web sites as: www.makemeheal.com. Many companies sell such products, and you may find others that you like.

Another wonderful resource is called "Look Good...Feel Better." It's a program designed to pamper you for hours while teaching you to modify your makeup to accentuate the positive about your changed body. You also get free cosmetic products and nail care since nails can become brittle from cancer treatment. Basically, you get a free, professional makeover! A make-up artist and cosmetologist improve your self-esteem and body image by transforming your looks. Many women find they feel lighter, happier, and more confident after this makeover. To find a provider in your area, go online at www.lookgoodfeelbetter.org.

If you have an ostomy bag that you'd like to keep discreet during intimate moments, try specially made lingerie that contains a pouch to hold and conceal your bag. Web sites such as www.wocn.org/patients/specialty_items.html and www.intimatemomentsapparel.com/firstpage.html offer unique garments with pouches sewn into the waistband that fully support the bag, but also conceal it from your lover. You may feel more free to express yourself sexually when wearing this type of lingerie.

Remember, you are more than an overweight or underweight body or a missing breast or uterus. The more you focus on your physical appearance, the more insecure you will become. It is important to stop doing whatever it is that compels you to feel badly

> *You are more than an overweight or underweight body or a missing breast or uterus.*

about yourself. Do you feel less attractive after reading women's magazines, or after shopping in the designer or junior sections of the department store? Stop doing whatever it is that makes you feel inadequate. If our value as women is solely dependent upon our looks, we are in trouble as a society. No doubt your accomplishments in your job, as a wife, mother, or partner more clearly reflect who you are as a person. Long legs, a nose job, and breast implants don't really tell us anything about the woman.

> *From birth to age eighteen, a girl needs good parents.*
> *From eighteen to thirty-five, she needs good looks.*
> *From thirty-five to fifty-five, she needs a good personality.*
> *From fifty-five on, she needs good cash.*
> Sophie Tucker, entertainer in the 1900s referred
> to as "The Last of the Red Hot Mamas"

Try to remember it is normal to change physically as we age, even without cancer treatment altering our bodies. On the positive side, if you have reconstructed breasts since cancer, your breasts will not be subject to the gravity pull that normally points aging breasts south; you're going to remain a perky woman.

Think about the potential benefits of your new look, no matter how outrageous, and write them down. Find humor where you can. Look at your list every day and say out loud, "I am beautiful, just as I am." Walk as slowly as you need to through your loss and grief, but also remember the new you is a pretty phenomenal woman.

A LITTLE HELPFUL INFORMATION...

Intimacy involves more than your body image. It involves how you feel about yourself, in total, and how you feel about a potential partner. Intimacy begins in the mind.

Debra Thaler-DeMers
as quoted on www.breastcancer.org

If you continue to have difficulty finding things you like about your appearance, then stop and write down everything you *don't* like about yourself. Is your negative body image simply a result of cancer? Could the way you feel about your body be influenced by more than cancer treatment? Do you recall whether or not your mother criticized her own appearance, or was she critical of your looks as a child? A long negative list usually means you feel quite insecure about your body image, which can lead to low self-esteem. You certainly don't need this added burden after cancer. If you find yourself with a long negative list, try this simple exercise by Carolynn Hillman:

Write down a list of your "fashion imperatives," such as "thighs should be firm and thin," "hair should be long and blonde." Write a list of "shoulds" and then compare this list with real women whom you find attractive. Finally, adjust your "shoulds" list to reflect the reality of women you believe are beautiful. Some may not have the thinnest thighs but radiate self-confidence; some may be older and still exude their sexiness. Another option is to think of women who are able to fulfill your "fashion imperatives" but are not attractive, in your opinion. Then decide for yourself who you would rather be.

It's also important to seek help if you feel low, sad, continue to grieve the loss of the old you, and can't find things about yourself that you like. See Chapter Six for a self-assessment quiz to determine if you might have depression. Depression after cancer is common, and it needs prompt treatment.

As If
by Kristen Spexarth

Somewhere along a lifetime most are broken
but we pretend we are not
taking up armor and masks
as if so doing we could fool the rest
as if a state of brokenness
was something to be ashamed of.
Contorted behind a smiling
and daily polished patina
we bend ourselves into pretzels for fear
a glimmer, warm and needing,
might shine through and blow our cool.
As if no one could read the details
running tickertape across our foreheads.
As if none could see our clumsy antics
tripping over bloated and rotting unattended business.
As if our single-minded hypocrisy
caused no pain.
As if we could hide from who we are,
as if who we are was hiding.
And still we are loved by those who see us
better than we see ourselves
love letting go of face forever and
taking up the heart of us
however broken.
Perhaps it is time to accept that broken is a part of place
that within these learning fields on earth
broken is a state of grace
wherein opportunity exists to learn the best
and the worst of it.
Perhaps it's time to recognize
and embrace the way we feel

picking our broken pieces off the ground of being
learning to knit them together again
with compassion for ourselves
larger than we were before,
larger than we ever imagined,
building with a new awareness
that somehow broken opens a door
invisible before.
And with newfound wholeness, expansive,
that embraces the broken and the mending
we become alive to the possibility
of sharing our humanity.

Unbroken we can never know this.
So let go of fear of falling,
stubbing pride and dignity
embrace the lessons a lifetime brings
laughing and crying wholeheartedly.
To ride our time without a bump
in our imagined being
would be to live an epoxy bubble,
brittle, indifferent, and unmoved by beauty
untouched by an ocean of love surrounding
beckoning us to jump.

Copyright © 2001 Kristen Spexarth
Reprinted with permission
From Passing Reflections
www.passingreflections.com

FACT OR FICTION?

"Anorexia nervosa exists in every country."

FICTION! This eating disorder is most common in countries where thin body types are preferred. In some countries, heavier women are seen as beautiful, and anorexia is rare.

"You are born with a sense of body image."

FICTION! Body image is learned and is connected to your self-esteem. It is about the way you perceive yourself based on emotion and imagination. A poor body image is not based on fact or the way others see you.

---

[1] Silver M (2004). Breast Cancer Husband: How to Help Your Wife (And Yourself) Through Diagnosis, Treatment, and Beyond, pp. 272–293. New York: Rodale, Inc. Emmaus, PA: Rodale Press Incorporated.

[2] Holzgang J. Facts on Body and Image. Just Think Foundation. Online: www.justthink.org/bipfact.html. (Accessed: December 3, 2001.)

[3] Olds T (1999). Barbie figure life threatening. The Body Culture Conference. VicHealth and Body Image & Health Inc.

[4] Field AE, Cheung L, et al. (1999). Electronic article: Exposure to the Mass Media and Weight Concerns Among Girls. Pediatrics, 103(3): e36. Online: pediatrics.aappublications.org/cgi/content/abstract/103/3/e36. (Accessed: August 11, 2006.)

[5] Women's Day and America Online (2006). Body Image Survey. Online: www.womansday.com/community/8189/body-image-survey.html?pl=. (Accessed: August 11, 2006.)

[6] Kilbourne J (1995). Slim Hopes: Advertising and the Obsession With Thinness [book on DVD]. Northampton, MA: Media Education Foundation.

[7] Dittrich L. About-Face facts on the MEDIA. Online: www.about-face.org/r/facts/media.shtml. (Accessed: August 11, 2006.)

[8] Cordova MJ, Giese-Davis J, et al. (2003). Mood disturbance in community cancer support groups. The role of emotional suppression and fighting spirit. Journal of Psychosomatic Research, 55 (461–467).

THREE

Self-Esteem: Me, Myself, and I

Self-esteem is when you compare your insides to somebody else's outsides.

Kevin Everett FitzMaurice

ancer can significantly affect your self-esteem. You might not always recognize the person staring back at you in the mirror. Confusion about who you are now, after cancer treatment, eventually seeps into your love life. Cancer influences the way you think and feel about yourself, and how you interact with other people.

As you already know, cancer can permanently change your appearance or the way your body functions (for example, survivors of colorectal cancer may need an ostomy bag for the rest of their lives). If you've had a gynecological cancer or chemotherapy for other cancers, you may not be able to have children after treatment. Some women who get cancer feel betrayed by their bodies and feel anger and hatred toward their bodies after treatment. This, too, significantly affects your self-esteem. And as Gloria Steinem says, "Self-esteem isn't everything; it's just that there's nothing without it."

You might be one of the fortunate women who emerge from cancer treatment emotionally stronger, feeling better about yourself, and respecting the strength you showed in coping with the whole ordeal. If you are one of these women, you have experienced what scientists call "post-traumatic growth." You have been able to find blessings in the ugliness of cancer. However, many women experience a loss of self-esteem while going through the diagnosis and treatment of cancer. Every time we must adjust to a crisis, our self-esteem is affected. It is understandable, then, if your self-esteem has taken a hit with your illness.

> *Many women experience a loss of self-esteem while going through the diagnosis and treatment of cancer.*

A healthy self-esteem indicates you have a well-adjusted, good opinion of yourself and your abilities. If you have positive self-esteem based on a true picture of your abilities and accomplishments, you will generally feel good about yourself and people will enjoy being around you. A healthy self-esteem is not the same as bragging about accomplishments, real or imagined; it is not boastful. A healthy self-esteem is appreciating who you are as a person.

> *If you put a small value on yourself, rest assured that the world will not raise your price.*
>
> *Anonymous*

Cancer can challenge any level of self-esteem, but it can devastate an already low self-esteem. If you were vulnerable before diagnosis, cancer treatment may only lower your self-worth. Once fallen, how do you raise that self-esteem, self-love, and self-confidence to a healthy level?

The first step is to find out exactly what you think of yourself. Morris Rosenberg is an expert in self-esteem assessment who developed a scale to measure levels of self-esteem.[1]

ROSENBERG SELF-ESTEEM SCALE

Circle your answers to the following questions:

1. I feel that I am a person of worth, at least on an equal plane with others.
    Strongly Agree   Agree   Disagree   Strongly Disagree

2. I feel that I have a number of good qualities.
    Strongly Agree   Agree   Disagree   Strongly Disagree

3. All in all, I am inclined to feel that I am a failure.
    Strongly Agree   Agree   Disagree   Strongly Disagree

4. I am able to do things as well as most other people.
    Strongly Agree   Agree   Disagree   Strongly Disagree

5. I feel I do not have much to be proud of.
    Strongly Agree   Agree   Disagree   Strongly Disagree

6. I take a positive attitude toward myself.
    Strongly Agree   Agree   Disagree   Strongly Disagree

7. On the whole, I am satisfied with myself.
    Strongly Agree   Agree   Disagree   Strongly Disagree

8. I wish I could have more respect for myself.
    Strongly Agree   Agree   Disagree   Strongly Disagree

9. I certainly feel useless at times.
    Strongly Agree   Agree   Disagree   Strongly Disagree

10. At times, I think I am no good at all.
    Strongly Agree   Agree   Disagree   Strongly Disagree

To determine your Self-Esteem Score (SES), assign a value to each question.

To questions **1, 2, 4, 6, 7,** the scores are as follows:

Strongly Agree **3**
Agree. **2**
Disagree **1**
Strongly Disagree **0**

To questions **3, 5, 8, 9, 10,** the scores are as follows:

Strongly Agree **0**
Agree. **1**
Disagree **2**
Strongly Disagree **3**

The higher your total score, the better your self-esteem.

No matter what your skills or role in life, you are valuable. To raise your self-esteem, you must truly understand your unique value, acknowledge that you are special, competent, important, possess good qualities, and that you are essential to this world. Self-esteem is just that: the way you perceive yourself.

> *Total self-esteem requires total and unconditional <u>acceptance</u> of yourself. You are a unique and worthy individual, regardless of your mistakes, defeats and <u>failures</u>, despite what others may think, say or feel about you or your behavior. If you truly accept and <u>love</u> yourself, you won't have a driving need for attention and approval. Self-esteem is a genuine <u>love</u> of self. Stop all adverse value judging of yourself. Stop accepting the adverse value judgments of others. Purge yourself of all condemnation, shame, blame, guilt & remorse.*
>
> *Author unknown*

Self-esteem problems begin in childhood. No surprise there, right? Perhaps you were fortunate enough to be raised by parents who showed you unconditional love. You'll reap the benefits as an adult as you'll be able to love yourself even when difficulties and challenges come your way. For those whose parents showed approval only when we met their expectations, we learn to look to others to find our value. Here is the beginning of years of self-esteem problems: when we believe we're only as worthy as others tell us.

DIFFERENTIATION?
Maintain Your Sense Of Self, Good Woman!

The man who trims himself to suit everybody will soon whittle himself away.

Charles M. Schwab

What can be done when we are taught as children to look to others for our value?

David Schnarch, a family and sex therapist, talks about the importance of "differentiation," which is the ability to maintain your sense of self when you are emotionally or physically close to other people. It's about being able to soothe yourself when you're feeling anxious without being swayed by other people's anxiety. He says that many of us rely on "borrowed functioning" to feel good; in other words, we rely on the way others view us to determine our own self-worth. In his book, <u>Passionate Marriage</u>, David Schnarch encourages us to appreciate our unique qualities, and to validate ourselves even when others are not kind or supportive.

> *As women, we especially live "in reflection," or are too concerned with what others think of us.*

As women, we especially live "in reflection," or are too concerned with what others think of us. We are too ready to please, and we too often adjust our behavior to be more acceptable to others. This is not a healthy way of functioning.

You will only have a healthy self-esteem when you realize just how important you are, without being influenced by what others think. We tend to value ourselves only for what we are good at. If we believe we are useless at something we think important, we feel inferior. On the contrary, if we think we are useless at a task we don't value, then we don't devalue ourselves by it because we don't care! For example, if I'm a bad housekeeper but I don't value a clean house, then the fact that I'm a bad housekeeper doesn't affect my self-esteem. On the other hand, if I do think an orderly house is important, I feel like a failure if I'm not good at it. Do you see? The value that you place on the skill that you either possess or lack contributes to your self-esteem.

SOLUTIONS FOR LOW SELF-ESTEEM
I Love Me, I Love Me Not

The living self has one purpose only; to come into its own fullness of being.

D.H. Lawrence

Now that you know *why* you have self-esteem issues, what can you do about these unhealthy issues?

First, find out on your own what you are good at. Everyone is good at something, so figure out your own gifts and talents. You may discover a new talent! It's common for people with low self-esteem to be very self-critical.

> *Everyone is good at something, so figure out your own gifts and talents.*

Do you think you are too critical of yourself? Ask, "If I knew someone identical to me, would I be as critical of her?" Chances are you would be much kinder when describing her, that imagined identical you. Remember the double standard? Well this is another example of it. If you are a person of faith, try imaging God telling you exactly what you are good at or what gifts you have been given for this life's journey. Don't be modest. Do be honest and positive when thinking about your own gifts.

Self-esteem is the belief that we are each worthwhile and have a contribution to make.

Gabrielle Bauer

Next, it's important to be around people who see the good in you, who encourage you to be kind to yourself, who help build you up. Avoid toxic people. Stay away from people who build themselves up by putting you down.

You are special, so treat yourself as if you were special. Be gentle, kind, and generous with yourself. Consciously drop the self-criticism. Learn to stop the negative thinking in its tracks, when you first hear the ugly voice of "I can't, I'm not good enough, I am inferior." Talk over it with "I can, I am, I will." Indulge yourself with a bubble bath, take up a new hobby, or treat yourself to a night out with good friends. You know how to "spoil" yourself, so just do it.

You have survived an extremely challenging illness, or are living with this illness, so pat yourself on the back for the way you dealt with it. Be your own best cheerleader.

Challenge those automatic thoughts, the habitual, harmful thoughts that lower your self-esteem. Replace these thoughts with a more positive, realistic assessment of whatever you are saying to yourself. If you still think you are no good, list the advantages and disadvantages of feeling this way. What are you getting out of this kind of negative self-talk? Resolve it quickly before this way of thinking becomes a habit.

If you need to jump-start your self-esteem, talking with a qualified counselor can help. A few sessions with a therapist who uses a technique called "cognitive behavioral therapy" can do wonders for your self-esteem. Cognitive behavioral therapy teaches you to change negative thinking patterns and replace them with new, healthy coping skills and ways of thinking.

If you are still not sure that you can improve your self-esteem, just take one small step in the right direction. Once you conquer that step, take the next. Before you know it, you'll be there, and we know you're worth it.

COGNITIVE DISTORTIONS
THROUGH THE LOOKING GLASS

But it's no use going back to yesterday, because I was a different person then.

Lewis Carroll, Alice in Wonderland

Thoughts are potent. No great thing was ever accomplished before it was a thought in someone's mind. There is power in your thoughts. The way you think about your love life after cancer will either improve your self-esteem or make it worse.

David Burns, a psychiatrist and top-selling author, describes ways of thinking, called cognitive distortions, which can make you feel unhappy or depressed.[2] It is tough dealing with a potentially life-threatening illness and treatment. Yet it is still important to try and think in ways that won't make you feel unattractive or sad. Do you have distorted thinking that is affecting your self-esteem and love life?

Take a look at some typical cognitive distortions or ways of thinking that you might have after cancer and its treatment.

COGNITIVE DISTORTIONS, CANCER, AND INTIMACY

1. ALL-OR-NOTHING THINKING: Your thoughts are totally negative. You believe you look "terrible" rather than "benignly imperfect" (like every other woman who is not a supermodel). Instead of acknowledging that your relationship(s) and sex life could benefit from some attention, you tend to think they are hopeless, and will soon be over.

2. OVERGENERALIZATION: Perhaps your first few sexual experiences after treatment were not pleasurable. You might now believe intimacy and sex will always be less unpleasant, and that you are powerless to improve either.

3. MENTAL FILTER: You focus solely on physical changes since treatment, such as a missing breast(s), a scar, or weight gain or

other effects of chemotherapy. These thoughts color your whole vision of who you are, how you appear, and the quality of your life. You may acknowledge that parts of your life are good, but you tend to concentrate on the bad.

4. DISQUALIFYING THE POSITIVE: Your husband or partner tells you that you look beautiful, that your missing or scarred breast doesn't matter, that YOU are all that is important. You hear this, but do not believe it. You think no one could find you desirable, and your partner is "just saying this to make me feel good."

5. JUMPING TO CONCLUSIONS: You interpret things negatively, even when facts don't support your negative conclusions.
    a. *Mind reading.* You just assume that others don't find you attractive or desirable without checking to see if this is true.
    b. *The Fortune Teller Error.* You are sure that telling your new boyfriend you had cancer will turn him off, or that a planned romantic evening will go badly because sex will be a disaster; so before you have even given the new boyfriend a chance to respond to your news, or begun your romantic evening, you have already decided that things will be terrible.

6. MAGNIFICATION or MINIMIZATION: You use the "binocular trick" to minimize your good qualities and focus on your bad. For instance, you focus on your mastectomy or lumpectomy scar(s) and "shrink" or undervalue your positive characteristics, such as being a warm, attractive, vibrant, and caring person. You develop the "double standard" attitude, or the tendency to be less sympathetic or tolerant of your own faults than you are of others.

7. EMOTIONAL REASONING: "I feel something, therefore it must be true." For example, since you *feel* undesirable or unattractive, you *believe* it must be true. You hate what the treatment for breast cancer has done to you, and feel unattractive, so believe you ARE unattractive.

8. SHOULD STATEMENTS: You try to motivate yourself with "shoulds" and "shouldn'ts," as if you first had to whip yourself into shape: "I should want to have sex" or "I should lose weight to be attractive." "Musts" and "oughts" are also offenders that usually make you feel guilty when you are using them on yourself. You can end up feeling angry, frustrated and resentful when you direct a "should" towards your lover, such as, "My partner should be more understanding that I am tired and not interested in sex."

9. LABELING AND MISLABELING: You label yourself as "used or damaged goods" instead of simply acknowledging your physical changes since treatment. This is an extreme form of overgeneralization. Also, when someone else's behavior rubs you the wrong way, you attach a negative label to that person. For instance, if you are irritated when your partner withdraws or on the contrary, becomes sexually demanding, you label your partner "a pain" or an "S.O.B."

10. PERSONALIZATION or BLAME: Personalization is when you blame yourself for something terrible another person has done to you. For example, if you blame yourself when your partner walked out on you after you told him that you had had cancer. Blame is when you accuse others of being uncaring when you are the one being unpleasant and treating them disrespectfully (even when you don't feel well!).

These ways of thinking, or cognitions, contribute to depression and low self-esteem. The way you talk to yourself is important. Do you think any of the following thoughts about yourself?

- "You idiot, why did you do such a dumb thing?"
- "I should be able to handle this better. What's the matter with me?"
- "I am sure that everyone knows that I've had cancer. Do I have a big 'C' written on my forehead?"
- "I hate myself, I think I look terrible, I'm 'damaged goods,' so why would anyone want to have a relationship with me?"

Your self-esteem, body image, and even the way you view your whole cancer experience is directly related to your thoughts. Women especially can end up with post-traumatic symptoms (such as reliving the cancer experience, or feeling fearful or irritable) after diagnosis and treatment. You may also wind up with a more positive perspective, called "post-traumatic growth." It's all about perspective and how you view the whole experience.

SOLUTIONS TO COGNITIVE DISTORTIONS

> *I wonder if I've been changed in the night? Let me think: was I the same when I got up this morning? I almost think I can remember feeling a little different. But if I'm not the same, the next question is, "Who in the world am I?" Ah, that's the great puzzle!*
>
> *Lewis Carroll, Alice in Wonderland*

Learning about negative thinking, or cognitive distortions, will help you recognize these thoughts as they enter your mind. You can change the way you think. You can also become more kind and gentle to yourself by acknowledging you might just be a little less emotionally strong than you were before cancer. Depression is common after cancer treatment, along with trauma and grief. (See Chapter Six for more information on depression and grief after cancer.)

When you feel unhappy, try to remember the particular thought you had just before this feeling. Identifying the thought or cognitive distortion that upset you can help change the way you respond to that thought. This will take some practice. An example:

> *A single woman says to herself, "No one will ever love me. I look awful, and I am damaged goods."*

First, identify the cognitive distortion, "No one will ever love me." This is "Jumping to Conclusions, Fortune Teller Error." Since no one knows the future, you can't know if this is true. Another example:

> *"I look awful."*

This is an example of "Mental Filter." You may truly believe you don't look as good as you once did, but cancer and its treatment can color your vision of reality. Even if you don't feel as good as before, it is unlikely that you look "awful." Are you starting to understand how to deflect these distorted thoughts? Here's another case in point:

> *"I am used goods."*

Can you guess which of the cognitive distortions this is? It's an illustration of "Labeling." You use emotionally charged words to describe yourself. Even if you feel that your scars or treatment impact your appearance, "used goods" has no real meaning for any person.

What are more rational responses to such thoughts? What truths can you respond with that make a lie out of the negative self-talk? Here is the distorted thought:

> *"No one will ever love me. I look awful, and I am used goods."*

The more rational response is:

> *"I am just as lovable as I was before I got sick. I have found love in the past so I will find it again. I may not **feel** as good as I used to, but I have been told that I look pretty good by people who have no reason to lie. 'Used goods' refers to things that are worn out, discarded, and of no value. Although I get tired sometimes, I do have value, and I don't feel like I should be put on the trash heap and discarded."*

Respond with rational, positive self-talk and you'll likely feel much better about yourself over time. Practice these skills and you will look at life differently and be equipped to rise above life's challenges.

Some women are truly traumatized by their cancer experience. If you think you fit this description, it's important to get in touch with other survivors to talk about it. Sometimes severe trauma such as war causes a condition called post-traumatic stress disorder (PTSD). An effective treatment used for people with PTSD is to review the experience and express feelings about the event, which allows the person to file the feelings into memory in a healthy way. The same kind of treatment may help get you through the trauma you felt with cancer.

During a crisis, we deal with what we have to cope with, almost instinctively, but we don't always process the emotional impact of what's happening at the time. You may start avoiding things that remind you of the trauma, such as not watching T.V. programs about cancer, or avoiding contact with others who have cancer. You do not have to dwell on your past experience; however, processing the fact that you had cancer might help you return to full functioning. Sometimes a professional counselor who practices cognitive behavioral therapy can help you through this process. Joining a survivors' group can also be helpful. Health professionals know that talking about your experience reduces the impact of the trauma.

> *During a crisis, we deal with what we have to cope with, almost instinctively, but we don't always process the emotional impact of what's happening at the time.*

Grief is another strong emotion that affects how you feel about yourself and your cancer experience. You lost some of your innocence as a result of the illness, and maybe your belief that you were invulnerable. It's possible you lost the ability to bear children. In order to move through grief, you have to acknowledge your losses, grieve them, and learn how to move forward. (See Chapter Six for more information on how to move past grief.)

It's also possible that since cancer, you are not just a survivor but a "thriver." Being a thriver means you were able to transcend the diagnosis and treatment, begin to live at a higher level, and more thoroughly enjoy your life. A thriver values every moment and is enriched as a result of this brush with mortality.

Each of us needs to feel good about ourselves just as we are. We are valuable simply because we exist. Making ourselves "smaller" or "invisible" so that others will feel "bigger" or "better" won't serve our purpose in this world...and we each do have a purpose. If you are person of faith, then you know that your Maker placed you here, not for you to hide your life but to live it <u>fully</u>. Once you understand that you are valuable, others will acknowledge it, too.

Finally, our self-esteem and body image are significantly shaped by our culture. Where did you grow up? What was your religion, your race, your value system, and what did your parents and culture teach you about sex, intimacy, and self-worth?

WHERE I COME FROM...
THE CULTURE OF CANCER

Cancer itself is a culture. When you become a part of cancer and a part of all those people involved in your cancer, such as your doctor, nurses, and social workers, you start seeing the world differently.
Subha Addy, MA, LCSW-AP, Oncology Social Worker

Your individual culture influences how you respond to cancer and its treatment. Culture can reflect your race, religion, personal values and beliefs, and what is considered "acceptable behavior" in your country of origin. As Subha teaches, "Culture comes from each of us. Each one of us is a cultural being. Our backgrounds teach us to see the world. It's not just about race or country, but culture is all about what and how we see the world."

Subha Addy is an oncology social worker who has cared for cancer patients at Sloan-Kettering and at M.D. Anderson Center and also in her own private practice. Subha also works with big companies educating employees about cultural differences for those leaving the United States on work assignments and those newly arriving in the United States. You could say that Subha is a cultural expert whose expertise also includes the culture of cancer. Subha says, "Cancer is a physical, cultural, emotional, and economic illness that affects the entire family and all who get involved with the patient. Culture provides the lenses through which we interpret our surroundings and act, react, and interact. We respond to cancer according to our culture. By culture I do not mean just race or ethnicity, which are only an aspect of culture, not the entire domain."

For instance, cultures greatly differ in the concept of modesty. Usually, non-Western countries are more modest. In fact, many Eastern cultures consider open expression of sexuality, especially by women, to be unacceptable behavior. For these women, talking about intimacy after cancer is inappropriate. In fact, simply talking about cancer may be improper. Because no one is talking about it, women either have no information or inaccurate information about cancer, its treatment, and side effects. Women can't talk about it, so they suffer. Myths and false information prevail.

A few years ago, the American Cancer Society University sponsored a course attended by health professionals from 32 different countries. During her attendance, and also throughout her years as an oncology social worker, Subha Addy has come across many myths from all over the world. Here are a few examples:

Armenia:	Cancer cannot be treated or prevented.
Chile:	Cancer is terminal and treatment is futile.
India:	It is due to fate. Nothing can help except prayers. It is due to some bad deed in the past.
South Korea:	Cancer is a death sentence.
Lebanon:	Cancer is a taboo subject. All cancer is fatal.
Malaysia:	Cancer is contagious, a source of shame; it is a punishment from God. Cancer treatment does not work.
Nigeria:	Cancer is due to witchcraft by enemies. It is incurable.
Pakistan:	Women who use contraceptives and/or do not breast feed get cancer.
Sierra Leone:	All illnesses are brought about by the devil as a form of Punishment.

In many countries where cancer is thought to be contagious, a husband will not come near his wife. This, in turn, makes the wife feel responsible for her cancer. She feels dirty or that she has done something wrong. As you can see from the common myths above, the blame is usually placed on the woman…as if having cancer wasn't enough of a burden.

As an example, a south Asian professor in a metropolitan city in the Mid-West who had breast cancer did not want her family to know about her illness, even keeping it a secret from her spouse. Her explanation was that she was worried that he would find her unattractive and not want to touch her in fear that the cancer was contagious. Her fears were based on the belief that a woman should be pleasing and attractive to her spouse, no matter what the situation.

Many cultures prevent women from talking openly about sexuality. In India, for example, "Modesty is an ornament that every woman should wear." It is difficult for women from such modest cultures to ask questions about intimacy after cancer. In fact, it is rude to discuss such matters with elders, including your mother or grandmother. Where can a woman with cancer turn to discuss such matters? It doesn't leave too many resources. If the sexual side effects of cancer treatment have significantly affected their intimate lives, sometimes the man will boldly ask the questions for his wife. If you live in a culture where you can freely discuss intimacy matters, count yourself lucky. The worst is that you will be embarrassed by asking the questions; the best is that you will get the help you need.

Cultures vary even within the same country. In the United States, for instance, there are many diverse ethnic, religious, and cultural beliefs. If you live in east Texas, you'll probably have different beliefs and values than someone who lives in northern California. Even in medicine, different cultures affect the way medicine is practiced. For instance, some states have significantly higher rates of back surgeries than other states. It appears that it is more acceptable to quickly proceed to back surgery to treat painful symptoms in some parts of the country. It's the same for treating cancer and the resulting side effects.

Your cultural beliefs about cancer can also affect the way you respond to cancer. As Subha says, "Culture makes a difference in people's attitudes towards treatment and therapy. Are you feeling guilty? Why are you feeling guilty? You didn't do this to yourself. Are people dying because they are not getting treatment? Cancer used to be a dirty word."

Such myths exist in more progressive cultures as well. For instance, a former common myth among African-American women in the United States was that African American women didn't often get female cancers, like breast or uterine cancers. Unfortunately, this kept many women from seeking regular cancer screenings. In some cases, medical treatment wasn't sought until the cancer was advanced. In Canada, young women overestimate their risk of getting breast cancer, while older women underestimate their risk.[3] Either way, the cultural myth kept both groups from getting annual mammograms to detect breast cancer. Education, even in industrialized, advanced countries like the United States and Canada, is key to changing inaccurate cultural beliefs. We hope this book dispels any inaccuracies you once thought true about intimacy after cancer!

Talking about sexuality and cancer is a difficult subject, irrespective of culture. Feelings of fear, pain, suffering, shame and guilt often make it a difficult subject to discuss openly. But there are exceptions, such as age, education, personality, positive self-identity, and information to name a few. The subject must be approached in an atmosphere of trust, which needs to be built up with care and over a period of time. Women often open up to another woman more easily than a man. Taking a cue from the individual and proceeding with caution is the key to approaching difficult subjects, such as cancer or sexuality. It is always good to ask the patient if there are certain areas that they would rather not bring up, and investigate what is the barrier. I have been successful in almost all cases to open up a meaningful discussion, given the time and genuine interest and treating the individual with dignity.

Subha Addy, MA, LCSW-AP

FACT OR FICTION?

*"A woman's sense of self-esteem and her body image
are totally independent of each other."*

FICTION! Right or wrong, a woman's self-esteem is strongly connected to her body image, especially in industrialized countries. We can break through this trap by teaching ourselves to focus on more important attributes and by fully understanding our value apart from our body shape and size.

"Parents are one of the strongest influences on our self-esteem."

FACT! Yes, this is true. Our parents' attitudes about our body's shape and size and our worth as a child greatly influence how we value ourselves as adults.

[1] Rosenberg M (1989). Society and the Adolescent Self-Image. Revised Edition. Middletown, CT: Wesleyan University Press.

[2] Burns, DD (1999). Feeling Good: The New Mood Therapy. Revised and Updated. NY: Avon Books.

[3] Institute for Social Research (2005). Study Finds Gaps in Breast Cancer Knowledge Among Ontario Women. York University. Online: www.cbcn.ca/en/?page=6765&section=4. (Accessed: August 11, 2006.)

FOUR

I'd Rather Read a Book

We were lying in bed one night a few months after my mastectomy but before my breast reconstruction surgery. I had just settled in to read a good book, glad for the quiet time and the opportunity to escape from reality. About then, my husband snuggled down into the covers and started creeping towards me. I knew what was on his mind. Not wanting to stop reading my book, I reached over to the nightstand, picked up my prosthetic breast, handed it to him and said, "Here honey, why don't you start without me."

Becky Olson, Cancer Survivor and National Speaker
(A fictitious story by Becky to illustrate humor in intimacy after cancer)

Is this a familiar story? It might help to know that you are not alone. You join a cast of thousands who are either going through cancer treatment or have come out on the other side only to find they don't have the same sensations, desires, or needs. Constant fatigue, along with other physical and emotional changes, may have left you wondering whether you would ever want intimacy again. More than half of the women treated for primarily female cancers report a significant loss of interest in intimacy. Many of these women ask: "How do I make myself care about having an active sex life again?"

If you are one of these women, don't despair! You can reclaim meaningful intimacy after a cancer diagnosis. Many women have been where you are now—not sure about the significance of sexuality in their lives since cancer. Once you received a diagnosis of cancer, your focus likely shifted from ordinary things to extraordinary efforts to save your life. Sex often falls to the wayside during the battle. As you move toward recovery and shift your thoughts toward returning to the "normal" aspects of daily living, you might find that your ideas about intimacy and sex have changed. It may take a little time for you to decide what you want in the future in an intimate relationship. Ultimately, only you will know what is satisfying now. No one else — not even your current lover — gets to decide that for you.

If you are unsure of what you want from an intimate relationship, reflecting on your present needs is a good place to start. You can also consider your partner's desires along with your own. Think about what you want from your partner. Do you simply need touching, hugging, cuddling, and holding for fulfillment? Do either of you want to go further with foreplay or sexual intercourse? If you are single, ask yourself, "What is it that I want from a future relationship? What kind of closeness will be most fulfilling?"

Intimacy comes from the Latin word meaning "inmost."[1] Intimacy is the sense of deepness and closeness you receive and give in your personal relationship; it includes touch and affection. Intimacy can also include the desire you feel for your sexual partner when intercourse is too painful or not possible. Intimacy includes the desire for inner closeness when physical oneness isn't possible.

On the other hand, "sex," as we know, can mean a lot of different things to a lot of different people, including a former American President! But for our purposes, the term "sex" will refer to the physical side of love making, including fondling, caressing, touching, oral sex, various kinds of foreplay, sexual intercourse, and orgasm. Sex is the physical aspect of making love.

The concepts of sex and intimacy may be confusing to you right now. Your brain or body may be saying one thing while your heart is saying another. While we all need touch and affection, how much you need is up to you. The way you feel about intimacy and sex now may relate to how sexually active you were before the diagnosis. If intimacy and sexual activity were important to you before cancer, it will likely be something you think about after cancer, even if you don't have the energy or desire to fully participate right now. If you were not sexually active before cancer, you may find it less important as you move into recovery and beyond. However, this doesn't mean that intimacy is not important for those of you less interested in having sex. It's possible to rekindle a love life, even if it was missing from your relationship long before cancer struck.

In fact, some women describe that after a cancer diagnosis and treatment, their sex lives actually improved! These women felt a renewed zest for life and expressed that enthusiasm through sexual contact and intimacy. They wanted to feel close to another human being and to feel united with the world; sex helped these women celebrate the fact they were alive.

MOTIVATION, SHMOTIVATION!

The last of the human freedoms is to choose one's attitude in any given set of circumstances, to choose one's own way.[2]

Viktor Frankl

In Man's Search for Meaning

The key to successfully reviving an intimate relationship is motivation. But how do you become motivated to reactivate your love life when you'd rather read a book; or when lovemaking or any form of intimacy holds absolutely no interest for you? For many women, this will be a conscious choice. You will choose to participate, not because you feel like it at the moment, but because you deliberately decide to renew this part of your life. The nature of your intimate relationship is a quality of life issue, both for you and your partner. However, you hold the power of choice. It will be important for you to decide when, where, and how you want to pursue intimacy, with whom, and what level of intimacy feels comfortable. You get to write your new sexual script. Do you want seduction, romance, lingering foreplay, with the lights on or off? When do you want to make love; in the morning or at night? Are you able to say, "no" to what you don't want to do?

We imagine you bought this book because you want to know how to improve your relationship with your partner. While we will give you the tools to help rekindle this part of your life, you get to decide what you want from your intimate relationship.

Since cancer, you may have changed the way you think about sex, or you may feel differently about your body (as discussed in Chapter Two). That is why it is important for you to begin thinking about your sexual script again; be willing to change it from what it used to be to what you now want and need. Intimacy in your relationship will likely make you feel loved, nurtured, and whole. Even though rekindling a fulfilling intimate relationship will take effort on your part, it will eventually be worth the effort you make, even if it simply helps you define what you want and don't want from your relationship.

Many women withdraw further into themselves after battling a life-threatening illness. It is an emotional roller coaster ride. The desire for touch might be gone, or so you think. If you fall into this category, rest assured that your physical and emotional desires can return with a little patience and motivation.

> *You may now look at lovemaking as "a chore" that you have to perform for someone else, like doing the laundry.*

Reclaiming a fulfilling intimate relationship will take some thought and effort. For women especially, remember that sexual foreplay begins in the mind. You may now look at lovemaking as "a chore" that you have to perform for someone else, like doing the laundry. Women can get into this rut even without being diagnosed with cancer. This is why it's important to consider what *you* want in the way of passion in your relationship. Again, intimacy is not just about having sexual intercourse; intimacy is about connecting with another human being. It's about kissing, touching, listening, talking, holding, hugging, longing, laughing, cuddling, lusting, and feeling close to the one you love. It's about you being pampered, stroked, honored, loved, valued, fulfilled, and satisfied. In fact, making love might be about everything else *but* sexual intercourse for a woman.

In order to enter into a gratifying sex life after cancer, you and your partner must openly communicate. This can be a little uncomfortable at first. If you haven't discussed sex in the past, it will not be easy, although it is not impossible to begin (see Chapter Eight to learn more about communication techniques). Learning how to effectively express your needs will be important, and this includes letting your partner know when you need to be left alone.

Marisa Weiss, MD, President and Founder of breastcancer.org and coauthor of <u>Living Beyond Breast Cancer</u>, puts it beautifully on the breast cancer support website www.breastcancer.org:

> *Sex and intimacy happen one step at a time. Give yourself time, give yourself love and affection, and make sure you give yourself credit all along the way for your hard work and courage.*

USE IT OR LOSE IT?

> *After his exam, the doctor said to the elderly man, "You appear to be in good health. Do you have any medical concerns you would like to ask me about?" "In fact, I do," said the old man. "After I have sex, I am usually hot and sweaty, and then, after I have it with her the second time, I am usually cold and chilly."*

After examining his elderly wife, the doctor said, "Everything appears to be fine. Do you have any medical concerns that you would like to discuss with me?" The lady replied that she had no questions or concerns. The doctor then said to her, "Your husband had an unusual concern. He claims that he is usually hot and sweaty after having sex with you the first time, and then cold and chilly after the second time. Do you know why?"

"Oh that crazy old goat," she replied. "That's because the first time is usually in August and the second time is in January."
(A widely circulated urban legend)

As you move through cancer diagnosis and treatment, thoughts of your previous sex life probably will begin to float to the surface. Because most of us really don't openly discuss our sex lives, you might wonder if sex after cancer is something you should be concerned about. The answer is an emphatic "Yes!" Intimacy and sexuality can make you feel more alive and connected to another human being than you have felt in a long time. If you ignore this aspect of your life, you could fall prey to the "use it or lose it" syndrome. Having sexual intercourse (or even masturbation) not only can elevate your mood and relieve pain, it will help maintain the tone and elasticity of your vagina. Similar to keeping your muscles strong through exercise, your vagina will stay in shape through sexual contact.

I think I might totally understand if my husband went out and had an affair. I look at him and remember being crazy about him and very turned on by him, but I can't seem to grasp that old feeling. It's like a switch was turned off.
Anonymous, Gilda's Club member

Many women voice this common, despairing story after cancer. In fact, one of the most universal complaints is the lack of sexual desire. Many factors reduce our sex drive or the need for intimacy. Both external and internal forces, such as the demands of daily living combined with the energy it takes to heal from cancer, can devastate a healthy love life. Cancer treatment is tough on the body. One doctor likens it to being hit by a semi-truck, and just when you think you're going to survive the effects of treatment, the heavy truck rolls back over your body. The physical side effects from cancer treatment alone can make having sex uncomfortable.

In addition, having cancer naturally gives rise to many raw, powerful emotions. Fear, anger, anxiety, sadness, and feeling out of control with your life are just a few prevailing emotions that you may have to process. Facing death and fighting cancer are not battles for the weak at heart. While we know that sex naturally moves down the list of importance when confronting cancer, the significance of intimacy should not be overlooked. Touching, kissing, hugging, and holding are still potent emotional and possibly physical healers, even during treatment.

Believe it or not, there are women who never stop wanting intimacy and sexual intercourse during treatment and recovery. We admire these women for their staying power; however, most women report a considerable loss of sexual interest after cancer treatment.

WHAT IF I'M (NOT) IN THE MOOD FOR LOVE?

It's as if I had a computer chip in my head that represented my former sex drive…it was removed along with the tumor.
Anonymous, Gilda's Club member

Intimacy and sexual problems are common after a cancer diagnosis. It is not "all in your head." What you're feeling is happening to thousands of other women. The lack of sexual desire often stems from a combination of both physical and psychological issues. Cancer treatments can change the way your body functions and responds, although many of these side effects are temporary

The longer you let intimacy slip from your relationship, the more time and effort it may take to reclaim the romance in your life.

and may slowly improve after treatment stops. If you are left with permanent physical and psychological changes, you can find new satisfying ways to express yourself sexually (see Chapter Seven for more information).

Physically, "feel good" chemicals (such as dopamine, endorphins, and adrenaline) are released into your body during lovemaking. These chemicals not only make you feel good but some are referred to as "bonding hormones" because they can make you feel closer to your lover. One of the substances, endorphins, acts like a painkiller. When endorphins are released into the blood stream, they naturally relieve pain. Additionally, these chemicals may help regulate mood and control your body's response to stress. The chemical dopamine can actually boost your mood and energy level. Orgasm, foreplay, and masturbation can activate these chemicals. So you see, lovemaking is far more important than just "satisfying an itch." It might be good for your overall well-being!

Psychologically, when you stop having sex, you may find yourself drifting away from your partner. A vicious spiral sets in. You and your partner are not intimate and may not be communicating about the lack of intimacy. Then it becomes increasingly uncomfortable to talk about the lack of sex in your relationship. Eventually, the result is complete embarrassment or discomfort in talking about not having sex, and the spiral goes on and on. The longer you let intimacy slip from your relationship, the more time and effort it may take to reclaim the romance in your life. If you wish to enjoy intimacy in your relationship, now is the time to embrace your partner, communicate your concerns, and rejoice in expressing your enjoyment for each other, both emotionally and physically, in whatever way you chose.

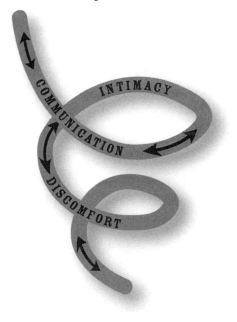

HEADLINE: SEX GODDESS RECONNECTS THE SENSORY NEURON

As we mentioned, there are many women who lose interest in sex after cancer treatment…and then there's Pam Bartholomew, RN. She is a champion in the pursuit of an active, healthy sexual life after treatment. In fact, there may be no woman more motivated to reclaim her love life. Sculptors would proclaim Pam the true "Sex Goddess," and the Venus Di Milo would learn from her. But Pam's desire and the reality of actually *having* an active sex life after treatment was a different story, even for someone as motivated as Pam.

Pam, a nurse who specializes in breast health care, found her own suspicious lump. At first, doctors were skeptical and didn't exactly share her concern. Intuitively, Pam knew better and kept insisting on a biopsy, which soon confirmed her worst fear: Stage 3 breast cancer. Treatment ensued, and so did the attendant physical changes, such as an extremely dry, thin, shrinking vagina and intense fatigue. These changes eventually led to one of her most momentous physical challenges. You see, Pam *loves* having sex with her husband. Pam is a true sexual gourmet. She was highly motivated to immediately return to an active sex life, unlike many of us who would rather "read a book." Pam is wonderful and unique, although not alone in her pursuit.

Being a nurse, Pam knew to ask for lubricants to alleviate a dry vagina and the other acute menopausal symptoms she now faced after chemo, radiation, and surgery. For weeks, she tried everything, including lubricating herself and her husband, trying different positions, and using a vibrator (we'll talk more about these options in Chapter Seven), all to no avail. Pam and her husband were successful in having other types of sexual intimacy, but they really wanted to enjoy intercourse again. It didn't look promising. But Pam is a tenacious woman who really wanted to make love to her dedicated husband. Finally, with a massive amount of lubricant, an anti-anxiety medication to relax, and careful positioning on top of her husband, Pam found success! And once that door was opened, so to speak, they were able to regularly enjoy careful, gentle intercourse.

You may ask, "Why was Pam so determined to have intercourse when it was so difficult?" Pam explains that she is crazy about her supportive husband. He attended most of her doctor appointments. He held her hand during chemotherapy. He was terrified of losing her. They fell in love in college and have been together for many years. Pam and her husband also love sex. Sex was a big part of their marriage before she was diagnosed. As we said earlier, if sex was important in your relationship before you got cancer, it will likely remain important after diagnosis and treatment. Because of her husband's support and love, Pam wanted to reach back to him in a way she knew he needed, and ultimately, that communication was through making love.

RETURN TO YOUR FIRST LOVE...

The first and most important step you can take in re-awakening your interest in intimacy or making love is to begin to think about it again. Remember, the biggest sexual organ a woman has is her mind. We need romance, tenderness, softness, and loving words to spark sexual interest, especially when it's been on the back burner for a while. We need to return to our first thoughts of love.

Think back about how you and your partner expressed love and intimacy with one another when you first fell in love. Were you playful or passionate? Try to remember how that felt...to desire and to be desired. As we mentioned before, intimacy is not just about the physical side of your relationship, but the physical side *is* important. What did you feel when your lover touched your hand or kissed you for the first time? What kinds of intimate moments have you shared over time, secrets that only the two of you know? Close your eyes and relive those memories. Think about how it would feel to reach out to your mate now, whether to kiss or hold hands or share a tender moment. That's intimacy. Return first to this emotional intimacy, and the rest will follow.

You can take it as slowly as you need, or change the way the two of you communicate closeness. The important thing is to reconnect that imaginary neuron in your brain that leads from your mind to the bedroom. Start talking about love and personal desires with your partner (see Chapter Eight for more information about communication). After cancer, the way you make love may change. What used to feel good before treatment may no longer spark a response or may even be uncomfortable now. Know that you can turn this new challenge around into an exciting adventure in finding out just what does feel good. Like Pam, you may have to work a little at having successful intercourse or to successfully engage in other types of lovemaking, but remember, just because you may have lost your breast or your uterus, doesn't mean you have to lose your love life or an intimate connection with another person.

When asked about how she finally succeeded in having sexual intercourse, Pam offered a few practical, motivational words of advice.

❖

PAM'S RULES OF ENGAGEMENT

1. Both of you need to approach sex with a good attitude, and draw on your sense of humor if possible.
2. Don't start too late in evening, i.e. it's important not to be tired!
3. Your partner must know that you are committed to making this succeed.
4. Fake it until you make it. Didn't you always want to be an actress on some level? (Pam advises that *telling yourself that you're interested in sex until you really are* can help.)
5. Use it or lose it, and if you lose it, you may lose the sweetest part of your marriage.
6. There is no such thing as too much lubrication. Get out the towels.

The longer you wait to engage in sexual contact (not just intercourse), the longer it may take to recover from physical symptoms and psychological detachment. In other words, "Use it or lose it."

For those of you still unsure about rekindling an active love life, give yourself permission to take it slowly. Think of restoring the passion like you're on a journey down an old, winding river that slowly flows into the ocean. You might actually enjoy a "cat and mouse game" of courtship to reawaken the emotional and physical sides of your relationship. A little playful exploration may help you discover new depths in your connection to your partner. Falling in love all over again, especially after a life-threatening diagnosis, may be deeper and more meaningful than anything you've experienced.

Many women who work through the loss of sexual desire after cancer may find their intimate relationship far more satisfying than before cancer. It's true! Treatment for common physical problems, such as a dry vagina and decreased libido, can make sexual intercourse more pleasant. Learning new ways to express yourself sexually can take the pressure off your old sexual script, and revive your relationship in ways you hadn't thought of before. Talking with the right doctor or a professional counselor who has experience with sex therapy about your symptoms and the way you feel about intimacy after cancer can help you to work through important concerns, validate your feelings, and teach you new ways to express intimacy. The loss of sexual desire does not have to be your new reality after cancer. Keep in mind, though, that deciding what you want from an intimate relationship after cancer can take some time, thought, and willingness to explore with your partner.

LOSS OF LIBIDO

How can I become sexual when the medication I am taking is such a passion killer? I'd rather clean the toilet than make love.

Celeste*, 43

A cancer diagnosis and its treatment can temporarily suspend your sex life. The severity of sexual dysfunction depends on the type of cancer and its treatment. As you probably already know, treatment can cause physical changes to your body. You may have already experienced hair loss, extreme fatigue, or mouth sores just to name a few, or more permanent physical changes, such as the removal of a breast or uterus. Cancer treatment doesn't exactly make you feel sexy. This is not to say, however, that intimacy will not remain important to you during and after treatment. You are a valuable, loved, and desirable woman with or without hair, breasts, or any other change to your body or soul.

PHYSICAL CAUSES OF LOST DESIRE

Surgery

Did you know that the nerve pathways that guide sexual function in women are not fully understood? These nerve pathways have been mapped out in men and are avoided during surgery to remove cancerous tumors from organs such as the prostate. But women's sexual nerve pathways remain a mystery. Our nerve pathways are not mapped nor spared during surgeries to remove cancerous tumors, such as hysterectomy, pelvic surgery, and oophorectomy (surgical removal of the ovaries). The result can be a loss of vaginal elasticity, increased pain during intercourse, inability to reach orgasm, and decreased lubrication and sensation during sexual activity. In addition, surgery that leaves you with an ostomy bag can make sex uncomfortable and awkward.

Chemotherapy

If you've had chemotherapy, then you already know it can wreak havoc on your sex life. Chemotherapy can interfere with hormone levels, damage ovary function, and cause premature menopause with symptoms such as hot flashes, vaginal dryness, loss of lubrication, and even problems with leaking urine. During treatment, the mucous membranes that line the vagina can become irritated, making the vaginal wall tissue paper thin and more likely to tear. Ouch! Painful intercourse is common after chemotherapy. This type of treatment increases your chances of developing yeast infections and sexually transmitted diseases, should you be exposed. Chemotherapy is a major cause of reduced sexual desire and the ability to respond to sexual stimulation.

Pelvic Radiation

Radiation for cancers in the pelvic area can lead to irritation and scarring of vaginal tissues, resulting in painful intercourse. While chemotherapy causes the vaginal wall to become thin, pelvic radiation can thicken vaginal tissues. A thick vaginal wall reduces elasticity, which makes intercourse painful.

WHAT SHOULD I EXPECT AFTER TREATMENT?

The vaginal muscles can lose elasticity after cancer treatment, making intercourse painful. The vagina may not produce enough moisture during foreplay, which further contributes to painful intercourse. You may need a great deal of lubrication to accommodate any kind of sexual contact. Fortunately, lubricants and other aids are available; but you have to ask the right doctor the right questions and spend a little time experimenting to see what works best for you. We will suggest products that you can use. This is also an area where you can do some "research" on your own to find what is most suitable for both of you.

> ❖ *The vaginal muscles can lose elasticity after cancer treatment, making intercourse painful.*

As mentioned above, radiation can cause the vagina to shrink. Some women need to stretch their vagina by inserting a vaginal dilator, which is a small tube usually made of rubber or plastic. Using a vaginal dilator or having sexual intercourse regularly, even once a week, can reduce the likelihood of tight scar tissue developing in the vagina, which makes intercourse painful. Of course, if intercourse is already painful, you can start by using a small dilator and then increasing its size over time until each size becomes comfortable.

The loss of libido and physical changes from treatment that cause lovemaking to be painful or uninteresting is common after many kinds of cancer treatment. In the beginning, a healthy sex life may not be a priority for you, and doctors who treat cancer will not usually ask you about the effects on your love life. Of course, when you receive treatment for cancer, there is nothing more important than saving your life. However, once you get through treatment, regardless of whether or not you are cancer-free, intimacy in your relationship will probably cross your mind. When you are ready to think about intimacy or sexual contact again, you may not know where to turn. Many women report that, when they finally were ready to talk about the effects of cancer treatment on their intimate lives, they were met with pats on the head from their doctors and told not to worry about it or were told that they were post-menopausal and that it should no longer be important to them! Worse, some women report the doctor was embarrassed by the conversation and provided no solutions or referrals for treatment. It is a private subject and some doctors are embarrassed themselves, but we have spoken to many doctors who were willing to talk about sex, including oncologists, gynecologists, and family doctors. We hope to spark a change by empowering you with the knowledge and tools you'll need to seek suitable care and reduce the unpleasant sexual consequences of cancer treatment.

IS IT ALL IN MY HEAD?

The answer is a resounding, "No, it is not all in your head!" Many women treated for cancer experience some level of lost libido or problems with painful intercourse, although for some, symptoms may be temporary. Recently, female cancer survivors were surveyed to identify sexual problems since being treated (often for breast cancer). The women who participated in three surveys were aged 20 to 70 years old, depending on the particular survey. Each survey reported similar results. More than half of the women who responded had a significant loss of interest in sex since treatment. The women also reported painful intercourse, perimenopausal symptoms (such as dry, narrow vagina and hot flashes) or worsening of existing menopausal symptoms. Few women said they were informed about the way cancer treatment would impact their sex lives or about the types of treatments available to resolve these issues.

Dr. Kydd conducted a survey of 300 women in the Saint John, New Brunswick, Canada area of women who had been treated for breast cancer in the last five years. Of those who responded, about one-quarter of the women were dissatisfied with their appearance since treatment. The dissatisfaction usually focused around removal of one or both breasts or around reconstruction surgery. One-third of the women had sexual difficulties or completely abstained from sexual contact since cancer. The primary issues were painful intercourse, a weakened vagina (atrophy), vaginal dryness, lack of interest in sex, and difficulty achieving an orgasm. An additional one-third of the women who responded said they were less interested in sex or had no interest whatsoever, and if they did take part, it was only to please their partners. In more than half of the women who participated in the survey, menopausal symptoms were either made much worse or suddenly appeared in young women after cancer treatment. More than half of the women said they had not talked to anyone about their sexual and intimacy issues since treatment. For the women who did get the courage to talk about these issues with their doctors, only half said the information provided by their doctor or other health professional was helpful.

Another survey taken by Educare, Inc. also asked women treated for breast cancer about the greatest impact to their sexual function.[3] The majority of the women complained of vaginal dryness and painful intercourse. Hot flashes, depression, weight gain, and insomnia were common. Many of the women had anxiety, a decreased sex drive, and difficulty reaching orgasm. About one-quarter of the women described body image problems, less energy, and mood swings. Some women had problems with anger and aggression since treatment. We wonder who wouldn't after battling cancer and then being left with these symptoms?

The Canadian Breast Cancer Network (CBCN) conducted a survey of young women (up to age 49 years) and rural women. It was presumed that most of the young women would have been pre-menopausal or not yet experiencing sexual menopausal symptoms, such as hot flashes and dry, itchy vagina, prior to cancer treatment. The CBCN found there was "utter silence" surrounding sexual dysfunction and how to understand the changes the women's bodies had gone through since treatment. One woman responded:

> "...(health providers) ignored my questions about sexuality and having children. They kept saying we would talk about that later on. Then menopause started and again, I was left on my own to learn about what was going on."
>
> *Anonymous*

After treatment, 96% of the women surveyed said they struggled with issues relating to their body image, including their physical appearance and sexuality.[4] Fertility after cancer treatment was a strong concern for many of these women, and they wished they had been better informed before treatment.

Sexual issues relating to cancer treatment are simply not yet given the significance they deserve. That's why we are writing this book! Your challenges with intimacy and sexuality after cancer treatment are *not* all in your head. As you can see, you share the same concerns as many other women. Now, the real question is, "What can be done about it?"

FIRST, A LITTLE OVERVIEW
A BRIEF LESSON IN SEXUAL ANATOMY

To really understand the changes in your body, you have to first understand the basic design of your body "down there." This information will also help you when you are ready to begin experimenting with your new love life (see Chapter Seven).

As women, we have sexual organs both on the inside and outside of our bodies. Our internal sex organs consist of the reproductive organs (ovaries, fallopian tubes, and uterus) and the vagina. Externally, we have the "vulva," which is a group of sexual organs that includes the vaginal opening, clitoris, mons pubis, and the labia majora and minora. The urethral opening is there too, but urine passes through this opening, and it is not considered a sex organ.

Internal and External Female Sexual Organs

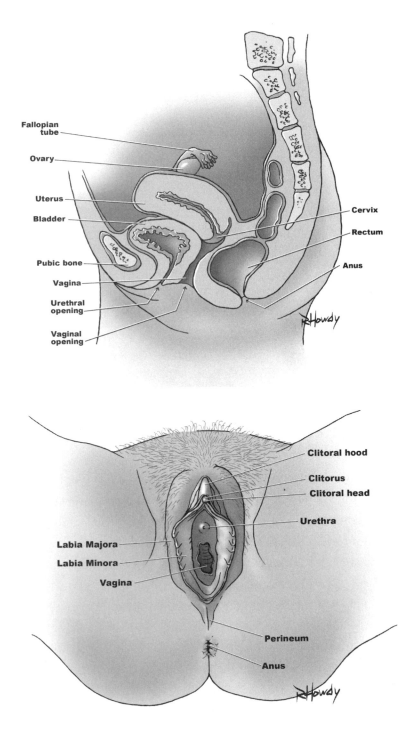

Some definitions:

- **Mons pubis:** The round, padded area that lies on top of your pubic bone and is covered with pubic hair.

- **Hymen:** The thin piece of tissue that partially blocks the entrance to the vagina.

- **Clitoris:** The clitoris is filled with nerve endings that respond to foreplay and sexual desire. It is sensitive to touch, and is the only true female sex organ dedicated purely to pleasure and not reproduction. The clitoris is shaped like a small button and is located where the two small lips (labia minora) come together. During sexual excitement, the clitoris is stimulated, fills with blood, and becomes erect, similar to a man's penis.

- **Labia majora:** The labia majora is known as the "outer lips." It's the large folds of skin that nearly cover up the rest of your external sexual organs. These outer lips are covered with pubic hair and are usually a darker color than the rest of your body.

- **Urethral opening:** This opening looks like a small slit and is located between the vagina and the clitoris. Urine passes out of your body through this opening.

- **Vaginal opening and vagina:** The vagina is a little over 3 inches (8 centimeters) long and begins at the vaginal opening. The vagina connects to the cervix, which then connects to the uterus. The walls of the vagina normally lie against each other; but when you are sexually stimulated, the elastic vaginal walls stretch to allow a penis to enter. If your vaginal walls lose elasticity and moisture and become paper-thin after cancer treatment, you can understand why having sexual intercourse can be painful or difficult. Without moisture and expansion of the vaginal walls to accommodate entry, the penis cannot glide into the vagina.

- **Labia minora:** This organ is referred to as the "inner lips," although the lips are still located on the outside of your body. The inner lips are not covered by pubic hair. The lips are a mucosal lining that shelters the front part of the vaginal opening. The inner lips are considered a sensitive erogenous zone. When you are sexually stimulated, they expand and turn bright red. This expanding organ usually stimulates the clitoris too. If you are unable to become sexually aroused from touching the clitoris, sometimes lightly touching the inner lips can help you reach orgasm more easily.

- **Perineum:** This is the space located between the vagina and the anus; it is made up of muscle and tissue.

- **Anus:** The anus is the opening that releases bowel movements; it is also made up of tissue and muscle.

The best way to get to a good look at your external sexual organs is to sit naked on the toilet or the edge of the bathtub and hold a mirror up to your vulva. You can use the definitions and graphics above to help you identify your own sexual organs. If you are uncomfortable looking at or exploring your vulva, you can learn from the graphics above, but we encourage you to march through your shyness and into the bathroom with a mirror. Remember Fannie Flagg's book, <u>Fried Green Tomatos at the Whistle Stop Café</u>, when the character Evelyn is trying to "find herself," so she attends a women's meeting where the women are instructed to undress, put a mirror to their vaginas, and "make friends" with it? Rest assured, you don't have to look at your vagina with a group or even by yourself if you don't want to. Still, we do hope you will spend some alone time getting to know yourself, and that the graphics help you identify the names of all your parts "down there."

COMMON SIDE EFFECTS OF TREATMENT

Breast, ovarian, uterine, cervical, and vaginal cancers all tend to cause the most sexual side effects, such as painful intercourse or a loss of sexual desire. However, other cancers, including bladder, colon, or rectal cancer, can also lead to problems with sexual function and lost interest. As you probably already know, the most common sexual side effects for women treated for cancer include:

- Loss of sexual desire and interest
- Difficulty becoming aroused or stimulated
- Dry vagina
- Thinning of vaginal wall
- Shrinking vagina or a clenching of the vaginal muscles (vaginismus)
- Painful intercourse
- Difficulty reaching orgasm

Diana Leitch, RN, RMT, compares the vagina and the vaginal opening (hymenal caruncle) to the rubber around the Mason jar lid. If the rubber lid dries out, it will become rigid and may crack or tear. The lid also won't seal properly if the rubber dries out. This is similar to the vaginal opening and walls. If there is not enough moisture, your vagina will dry out, become paper-thin, and lose elasticity. Touching or having any kind of sexual contact will be uncomfortable or even painful. The vagina must be kept lubricated even when you are not having sex.

In addition to the physical side effects from cancer treatment, it is also common to pull back emotionally from your partner after treatment. The reasons vary, but often, you withdraw because of physical or psychological pain, such as being nauseous,

Don't be too quick to dismiss the value of intimacy and healthy sexual contact in your cherished relationship.

tired, depressed, or anxious. You may simply be too tired to connect with your partner. What is important to understand is this: It is normal for you to feel this way after cancer. Even women who have not had cancer sometimes struggle with these issues, and these women don't have to contend with the additional demands of healing from cancer and its physical and psychological consequences. It's totally understandable if you are not interested in intimacy or sex at the moment! If this was an important part of your life, it is possible that you can recover from many side effects and go on to enjoy a happy, healthy love life. You may be able to enjoy your sexual relationships more than ever and experience more satisfying sex than before cancer.

If you have attempted to reach out to your partner sexually but were prevented due to pain, seek treatment from your doctor. This type of pain can occur as a result of hormonal changes, a decrease in the production of moisture in the vagina, and from scarring or a change in the size of the vagina. Treatment is available for all of these common complaints, so be sure to check with your doctor.

If you continue to have little or no interest in sex or even intimacy, and if sex was important to you or your partner before, and you would like it to be again, it's important to seek help to sort it out. There are many ways to reawaken this side of your life. Remember the importance and value in feeling connected to your partner, for both of you. There are physical consequences in prolonging the loss of sexual contact – the "Use It or Lose It Syndrome" is real. Even if you think you could never be interested in intimacy or making love again, or if you have been repeatedly unsuccessful at your attempts, this doesn't mean it will always be this way! Don't be too quick to dismiss the value of intimacy and healthy sexual contact in your cherished relationship.

OH GOODY...EARLY MENOPAUSE!

Some cancer treatments, such as treatments for breast cancer and cervical cancer, can lead to symptoms of premature or sudden-onset (acute) menopause. This means that your body "suddenly" goes into menopause, causing sometimes severe, abrupt symptoms normally associated with menopause, such as hot flashes, night sweats, and an extremely dry vagina. Chemotherapy and radiation therapy can alter your normal hormone levels. A loss of hormones such as estrogen or androgen can trigger hot flashes, make the vagina dry and tight, and decrease your desire for sexual pleasure. Hormone replacement therapy can help, but few women can safely take hormones after female cancers. If you've had a cancer that was hormone-sensitive, hormone replacement therapies may not be a safe option as they might stimulate the spread of the cancer. Other helpful treatments are available, however, and are discussed in the "What Can Be Done" section of the next chapter.

Some women complain they can't reach orgasm after cancer treatment. Usually, this is due to painful intercourse. Trying different positions might relieve the discomfort, or having "outercourse" where the penis does not penetrate the vagina can also be satisfying for many couples, especially while your body is healing. Learning to explore your new erogenous zones may also be effective and is discussed more fully in Chapter Seven. Sex can be better than ever, and orgasms definitely do NOT have to be a thing of the past.

If you now have an ostomy bag after cancer treatment, sex and being naked in front of your partner can be awkward at first. The bag may leak, give off an odor, be in the way, or be uncomfortable when attempting sexual contact. You may be self-conscious of the bag and unsure how to "ignore it" when trying to make love. You may avoid taking your clothes off in front of your partner. Rest assured, there are solutions! You, too, deserve a healthy, active love life. You may have to change your sexual script, the way you made love in the past, but desire, intimacy, and pleasure are still possible.

FACT OR FICTION?

"Sex drive disappears with chemotherapy."

FICTION! Fatigue and other side effects from chemo can greatly reduce interest in sex, but doesn't have to completely disappear.   Don't forget about Pam's Rules of Engagement!

---

[1] Hoad, TF, ed. (1986). Concise Oxford Dictionary of English Etymology. Oxford, England: Oxford University Press.

[2] Frankl V (2000). Man's Search for Meaning. Boston: Beacon Press.

[3] Kneece JC (2002). Sexuality After Breast Cancer Treatment. Focus Group Study Results. Educare Inc.

[4] Canadian Breast Cancer Network, Ontario Breast Cancer Community Research Initiative (2003). Nothing Fit Me: The Information and Support Needs of Canadian Young Women With Breast Cancer. CBCN Final Report.

FIVE

Reading the Right Book

WHAT CAN BE DONE?
SOLUTIONS TO COMMON PHYSICAL SEXUAL PROBLEMS

*Y*ou've already seen that as a woman, your sexual "wiring" is elaborate. It's a complex interaction between the physical, psychological, and communicative sides of your life. A man's sexual function is much more simple.

MEN

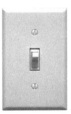

WOMEN

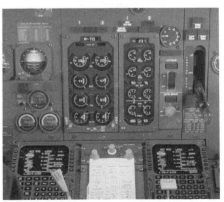

As the illustration shows, a man basically has an on/off switch when it comes to sex. A woman, however, has an entire system of knobs, valves, levers, and switches that function at various levels. The parts must be lubricated, coaxed, touched, and turned on in the right order or she will experience "system failure." Adjusting knobs and determining the order of the "ignition sequence" can take some time and exploration, and it may have changed since cancer. What worked for you before you were treated for cancer may not work now. If your breasts were an erogenous zone before cancer, you will need to find a new erogenous zone if they have been removed or altered. If you were the one to initiate sex or intimacy before cancer but now have little or no interest, your partner may need to learn to gently make the first move (see Chapter Eight on communicating for more information).

CAUTION

The recommendations presented in this chapter and throughout this book are merely suggestions. Remember to practice safe sex and to be careful when exploring new erogenous zones. Your body is more fragile, your immune system may have been weakened through chemotherapy, and you may be more susceptible to infections. Thin vaginal walls put you at greater risk for increased bleeding and resulting infection. Check first with your health professional about your own personal potential risks.

PROBLEM: No sex drive. Might not care about ever having sex again.

SOLUTION: Identify when you are least fatigued, and schedule alone time with your lover. Know your medication side effects. Have hormone levels tested. Rule out depression or other illness, such as thyroid problems.

The loss of sexual desire after cancer is both a physical and a psychological issue. Let's first talk about the physical solutions for this loss, and then we'll discuss the psychological solutions further below.

The loss of interest in sex and intimacy is not just imagined. It's not simply an "attitude problem." It's a very real biological reaction to the chemicals used to kill the cancer in your body. Decreased sexual interest is also a common side effect of some prescription medications, such as high blood pressure medications. You can lose interest in sex if your hormones are out of balance. In addition, lost desire can result from the incredible fatigue that accompanies cancer treatment. Desire can be lost when you are out of practice. For most people, sex moves down the list of importance after a cancer diagnosis. It's possible, however, that if you don't intentionally move it back up the list, a new habit will form: The habit of not making love.

THE FATIGUE MONSTER

Physically, it is important to tackle the issue of fatigue first. Are you getting enough sleep? Are you getting enough help for daily activities, chores around the house, and the demands of your job? If you think you could use more help...ask for help. As women, we multitask. We also have a tendency to become martyrs.

> *Christine* wanted to protect her husband and children from the stress of her cancer diagnosis and treatment. She tried to shield her children by making sure their lives continued as normal. Christine was a typical soccer mom who drove her children to all school and after school events. She made sure they did their homework, took their baths, and felt nurtured and loved.*

Christine tried to keep this level of activity up shortly after surgery and throughout her chemo treatments. Her husband assumed she was feeling well enough to do it all. Her friends saw her at soccer games, and commented on how good she looked. The only way Christine didn't crash and burn each day was to sneak in a 30-minute nap before the kids got home from school. She was in bed – asleep and not having sex – by 9:30 every night.

Recovering from cancer is a team effort, especially if you are caring for others. If your children are old enough to help out, assign some household chores to them. You also have to surrender perfection…if it's not important, then let it go. If you can afford to hire someone to do the housework, do it. If you have friends who have offered to help out by cooking, cleaning, or watching your children, take them up on it! If co-workers have offered to take some of your projects, let them; if they haven't, then ask them to do so. Lighten your load, even if you are months past completion of treatment. It doesn't matter that others think you should be well enough to handle all of your obligations on your own. You, and only you, know whether or not you are too fatigued to fully function. If you continue to experience the kind of fatigue that interrupts your intimate life, it is a problem. Ask for the help you need. Then focus on you, your love life, and what you want from it.

Recovering from cancer is a team effort, especially if you are caring for others.

Next, determine if there is a particular time of day and certain days during the week when you have more energy. Do you feel most rested first thing in the morning? Do you feel less tired after the luxury of an afternoon nap? Identify when you have the most energy during your day or week. Then schedule some alone time with your mate during that particular time. Eliminate all distractions. If you have to meet at a hotel, then do it. Even if you do not have intercourse, spending that time together getting naked, stroking, snuggling, hugging, kissing, petting, and loving each other is imperative to rekindling your sexual interest. You may even simply enjoy lying close together fully clothed or talking softly about your relationship. Your lovemaking journey might begin again merely by spending time alone together talking.

This scheduled rendezvous is the perfect time to begin communicating about what each of you now wants from your love life. Be mindful that your erogenous zones may have changed. After you've read Chapters Five through Eight, you will have the tools you need to communicate your desires and to explore new sensual triggers. You don't have to figure it all out during your first tryst. In fact, you may soon begin to look forward to these "dates." It's important to schedule time when you have energy to devote to the well-being of your physical and emotional relationship with your partner. Be flexible and meet when you know you feel your best. You might be surprised that you soon look forward to this time alone with your lover, even if you are not yet having sex.

MEDICATIONS, ILLNESS AND SIDE EFFECTS

Many types of medications, both prescription and non-prescription or over-the-counter (OTC), can reduce your interest in sex. Antidepressants, high blood pressure medications, sedatives, pain killers, drugs for nausea, cancer medications (such as tamoxifen), and even decongestants can reduce libido. Weight loss drugs (anorectics), heart medication, hormone therapy, and even cold medications can also affect your sex drive. Talk with your doctor if you feel that one of your medications might be causing your loss of libido.

If you are taking any medications, it is important to know the possible side effects of each medication. You might want to read all of the packaging or prescribing information carefully for any medication or even herbal therapies you are taking. Talk with your doctor about the potential sexual side effects of any medications you are taking; some OTC medications can also affect your sex drive.

If you do experience loss of libido while taking a medication, it is possible another medication may be available that will not cause these side effects. However, if you must continue with a particular medication that decreases your sexual interest, you can still enjoy an active love life, although it will take a little more effort. It might help to schedule your intimate time when the medication is at its lowest strength. Your doctor can help you determine when that is and provide other kinds of related information. Don't be afraid to ask for possible alternatives if you have lost interest in sex as a result of taking medications. It's important to learn what you can do to bring back your sex drive physically and emotionally. Your life is not just about trying to survive – sex impacts the quality of your life.

Certain chronic illnesses can also reduce your sex drive. Heart disease, diabetes, and hormone imbalances are all associated with decreased interest in sex. Schedule an appointment with your doctor to find out if your decreased sexual desire is caused by another illness. Treating the associated condition can resolve or reduce your symptoms. For instance, if you have a sluggish thyroid, you may feel tired and depressed. Treating this condition can revive your energy level and consequently, your sex drive, so check with your doctor.

> **PROBLEM:** *Symptoms of menopause: hot flashes, dry vagina, tight or narrow vagina, thin vaginal walls, and painful intercourse.*

> **SOLUTION:** *Lubrications, vibrators, vaginal dilators, Kegel exercises, and a good relationship with your gynecologist or primary physician.*

First, it is very important to establish a good relationship with either your family doctor or your gynecologist so that you feel comfortable talking about your sexual concerns. It is also important that you receive good information. If your doctor is not able to help you, consider getting a second opinion. Finding the right, qualified doctor is invaluable to your becoming sexually healthy again if you have experienced severe or abrupt menopausal symptoms after cancer. Fortunately, there are some wonderful health professionals out there willing and able to help you through these issues.

HORMONE THERAPY

*My vagina was so dry and tender; it felt like sand paper or like
it would split if I bent down.*

Linda*, 52

When a woman approaches menopause naturally, losing interest in sex can be a common problem. She may choose, with her doctor, to begin taking low doses of hormones to relieve symptoms such as hot flashes, and a dry, itching vagina. A low level of the hormone testosterone in a woman's body may result in lost desire. (Testosterone, a predominately male hormone, does exist at lower levels in a woman's body.) If you develop sudden or aggravated symptoms of menopause from cancer treatment, using hormones to treat your symptoms may not be an option for you. Any kind of hormone therapy may be risky, especially if you've had a hormone-sensitive cancer.

Nevertheless, using hormones after a hormone-sensitive cancer is an individual choice. If your menopausal symptoms are severe, a low-dose hormone therapy may be an option. Dr. Eshwar Kumar, Head of the Department of Oncology at the Atlantic Health Sciences Corporation in Saint John, New Brunswick, Canada, responds to this concern by saying, "Years ago it was taboo to suggest that a patient use hormonal creams with breast cancer. However, quality of life is a huge issue. The discussion about using estrogen after cancer should be individualized to the patient, and center on her history and the severity of her symptoms. A woman needs to be informed about the risks of using low-dose estrogen creams. However, if she's having severe menopausal symptoms that interfere with the quality of her life, the benefits of using a low-dose estrogen cream might outweigh the risks. A patient may choose to use low-dose estrogen after a discussion with her doctor, especially if she had a low-risk breast cancer many years ago. The important thing is that she makes an informed decision."

If the quality of your life is in jeopardy because of severe menopausal symptoms, talk with your doctor about your personal risks of using hormone therapy. Then you can make an informed personal decision as to whether or not hormones are right for you. If hormones are not an option, there are still other ways to reduce your symptoms and increase your desire.

There are three basic types of estrogen: Estradiol, which is easily absorbed by the body and, therefore, the most potent and dangerous form to use after a hormone-sensitive cancer; estrone, which absorbs into the body more slowly; and estriol, which the body only absorbs minimally. Estriol may be less risky for a woman who has had breast cancer than other forms of estrogen, especially estradiol, but that doesn't mean it is necessarily safe for you to use. Further research is needed to determine whether estriol, even in a "natural" form like a soy compound (also known as a "phytoestrogen"), is safe for you to use after having a hormone-sensitive cancer. It's a good idea to discuss with your doctor the use of any type of estrogen (including holistic or herbal products that contain natural estrogens) before you decide whether to take it.

After speaking with your doctor, it's possible he or she may prescribe low-dose, localized hormone medications (such as a vaginal cream) to help make sexual contact more comfortable. For example, the Estring is a plastic ring filled with estrogen that is placed into the vagina. The Estring can thicken and lubricate the vaginal walls, but it's possible that your body might absorb some of the estrogen. Another estrogen-based treatment is estradiol vaginal tablets, such as Vagifem tablets. These tablets are inserted into the vagina regularly to relieve symptoms such as dry, itching, and sore vagina. However, if you've had an estrogen-sensitive cancer, you may not be able to use an Estring or vaginal tablets to relieve dryness. By introducing more estrogen into your body, you may stimulate the return of cancer cells. Using a hormone treatment like an Estring is a personal choice that you make with your doctor after discussing all of the risks and the severity of your menopausal symptoms.

Dr. Mary Beth Harman, an OB/GYN and sex counselor with Women's Health Care of Trumbull, Connecticut, explains that while not all primarily female cancers are hormone-sensitive, the risks between hormone therapy and cancer are still not clear. For example, the use of testosterone to increase libido or energy levels after a hormone-sensitive cancer may be risky due to the body's ability to convert testosterone into estrogen. If your menopausal symptoms after cancer treatment are severe, talk to your oncologist or OB/ GYN to find the best solution to ease your discomfort.

OTHER MEDICATIONS

If you are nervous about attempting intercourse, especially after a painful sexual experience, your tense muscles can make lovemaking difficult. You will not be aroused or interested in making love if you think it is going to be painful; in fact, you'll avoid it, and who wouldn't? Sometimes an anti-anxiety medication, such as alprazolam (Xanax), can help you relax and allow a more pleasant experience during lovemaking. Another option is to use a muscle relaxant, such as cyclobenzaprine (Flexeril) or metaxalone (Skelaxin). Be aware, however, that these medications can be habit-forming and may worsen symptoms of depression. Ask your doctor about these medications if you think relaxing tense muscles or reducing anxiety would help you succeed at resuming your sexual life.

Loss of sexual desire is a complex issue. It's not always due to one thing, such as a decline in hormone levels, menopausal symptoms, or psychological concerns. It is a combination of all of these issues and more. For instance, if you are a woman in menopause, your husband is likely experiencing the effects of aging as well. Perhaps he has difficulty getting or maintaining an erection. Combining his issue with your possible symptoms of menopause (dry, tight vagina), can make having sexual intercourse a challenge. Your partner may also be fearful of hurting you since you had cancer and may be holding back.

Dr. Harman explains that after radiation and chemotherapy, the vagina's capacity to repair itself can be substantially diminished. The elasticity and lubrication is lessened, making penetration potentially painful and difficult. That is why it is important to rewrite your sexual script or the way you make love, to include gentle and careful sexual contact after such cancer treatments.

YOUR NEW MANTRA:
LUBRICATE, LUBRICATE, LUBRICATE!

Remember Pam's sixth rule of engagement? She is right. A good vaginal lubrication can do wonders to ease the discomfort of intercourse when your body is no longer producing enough vaginal moisture. If a lubricant helps you enjoy pain-free sexual intercourse, you are likely to be less anxious the next time you are intimate with your partner. When your muscles are not as tense, intercourse will be more enjoyable. There are basically two types of vaginal lubricants that may be safe for you to use if you've had a hormone-sensitive cancer: water-based and oil-based lubricants.

Some of the most commonly used lubricants are *Astroglide, Today, Moist Again, Probe, K-Y, Surgilube, Women's Health Institute's Vagi-Gard,* and *Bag Balm.* You can pick these up at your local drug store, your doctor's office, or by ordering online.

WARNING

Only use a water-based lubricant if your partner is using a condom, because other lubricants damage condoms. Oil-based (petroleum and silicone) lubricants also stain sheets, so you might want to have towels handy if you decide to use an oil-based lubricant.

Before having sexual contact, spread lubricant liberally over and inside your vagina, over your labia, clitoris, and on your partner's penis, fingers, and whatever will come in contact with your vagina. If you find you need a significant amount of lubrication, you can apply it internally using surgical gloves. You might want to keep a tube in your bathroom and near the place(s) you usually enjoy intimacy. You can even use the lubricant during foreplay if your partner is willing.

Vaginal moisturizer:

A product called *Replens* is often used to increase vaginal moisture. It is estrogen-free, so it may be okay for you to use if you've had a hormone-sensitive cancer. *Replens* is not a lubricant but is an over-the-counter (nonprescription) moisturizer that works by helping the vaginal wall hold water. Over time, *Replens* will thicken the vaginal wall tissue and make intercourse more comfortable. Check with your doctor to see if this type of product is right for you.

Water-based vaginal lubricants:

Most vaginal lubricants are water based. They are considered safe because they are easily washed from your body. There are a variety of choices of water-based vaginal lubricants that come in various consistencies from thin to thick. A thicker lubricant may stay on longer and create an extra cushion of comfort. Some women prefer a thinner lubricant that feels more like their own body's lubrication. Just choose the consistency that feels right and works best for you.

Examples of water-based vaginal lubricants on the thin side are *Astroglide*, *K-Y*, and *O'My*. In fact, *K-Y* has come out with a warming *K-Y* lubricant that some women find soothing and erotic. However, if one of your symptoms is a feeling of burning during intercourse, then a warming lubricant may be a bad idea for you. Medium consistency lubricant product examples are *Slippery Stuff* and *Liquid Silk*. Thick and jelly-like lubricant product examples are *Maximus* and *Astrogel*. An example of a very thick and stringy lubricant is *Probe*. You may want to choose the lubricant based on the severity of vaginal dryness: the dryer your vagina, the thicker the lubricant needed. Thicker lubricants may also be more helpful when using sex toys or vibrators, although a thicker lubricant is not necessary for successful use of toys or vibrators. Also, water-based vaginal lubricants can sometimes dry a little "sticky" or "tacky." You'll probably need to reapply the water-based lubricant a few times during lovemaking as it can dry out. Besides, using a lot of lubricant may help you succeed with intercourse if this has been a problem.

Water-based lubricants sometimes contain preservatives that can cause allergies. If you have sensitive skin, you may want to try a lubricant that does not contain preservatives, such as *O'My* or *Probe*. If you are prone to yeast infections, you may want to select a lubricant that does not contain glycerin, such as *Liquid Silk, Maximus,* or *Slippery Stuff*. It may take a little experimentation to find out which lubricant works best for you. Companies often give away samples of their lubricants on their Web sites, in your doctor's office, or at adult sex toy stores.

Oil and silicone-based vaginal lubricants:

All oil and silicone lubricants are thin and slippery, unlike water-based lubricants. Oil and silicone-based vaginal lubricants also last longer than water-based lubricants, so you don't have to reapply the lubricant as often. Silicone and oil-based lubricants don't usually cause allergic reactions, so they are a good choice if you have sensitive skin. You can also use them as a body massage oil for both you and your partner during foreplay. One drawback of silicone and oil-based lubricants is that they are difficult to wash from your sheets, so you may want to use towels. They are also more expensive than water-based lubricants, although you may have to use less of the silicone and oil-based lubricant for the same effect.

There is not much difference between the types of oil-based vaginal lubricants except that the best quality brands use a dense ingredient called dimethicone, which is what makes them more expensive. Some women say this ingredient feels more silky and luxuriant than the brands made without it. Examples of oil-based vaginal lubricants that contain dimethicone include *Eros* and *Wet Platinum*. An example of a basic oil-based vaginal lubricant is *ID Millennium*.

If you've had difficulty having intercourse due to a dry, tight, or thinning vagina since cancer, use a large amount of lubrication, both on yourself and on your partner's penis before attempting intercourse. You may need to reapply the lubrication during foreplay, depending on how long foreplay lasts and the type of foreplay you're enjoying. If you are experiencing any menopausal symptoms, get acquainted with a good vaginal lubrication before you return to making love. Lubrication can enhance your sensuality, sensitivity, and make lovemaking more fun, especially after cancer treatment.

AND STRETCH...AND TONE... VAGINAL AEROBICS?
KEGEL EXERCISES

Some experts think that learning to squeeze the pubococcygeus or "PC" muscles located in the lower third of the vaginal canal (known as "Kegel exercises") will strengthen and tone the muscles of the vagina, which may help a woman reach orgasm more easily. Kegels increase blood flow to the genital area and can assist in sexual arousal. They are essential in treating some types of vaginal shrinking and when using vaginal dilators. Kegel exercises can also prevent certain problems associated with aging, such as urinary incontinence.

The best way to "find" your PC muscles is to stop urinating in mid-stream. The muscles you used to stop urinating are the PC muscles. Now that you know where they are and what it feels like to squeeze the PC muscles, try squeezing them (on an empty bladder) up to 3-5 seconds, releasing, and then repeating. Repeat the squeezing and relaxing cycle at least 10 times. Because no one can tell when you are doing Kegels, you can do them anywhere: shopping, sitting at work, standing in line, or whenever you think about it. Practice doing Kegel exercises throughout the day, trying to increase the amount of time you squeeze the PC muscles and the number of times you do them.

THE SHRINKING VIOLET...I MEAN VAGINA?

In response to some cancer treatments, especially pelvic cancers, the vaginal opening and base of the vagina will become narrow and tight; this condition is called vaginismus. It is nearly impossible or extremely uncomfortable to have sexual intercourse and some types of foreplay.

Lubrication alone probably won't be enough to conquer this issue. A common solution is to use a vaginal dilator. Your doctor can prescribe a vaginal dilator kit or you can obtain one online at websites such as www. vaginismus.com/products/dilator_set/

Check with your doctor first before trying a vaginal dilator. You don't want to worsen an existing medical problem by using a dilator, especially if you had pelvic radiation or surgery. Vaginal dilators are usually made of plastic or latex and come in a set with a range of sizes. It is important to schedule about 20 to 30 minutes of private, uninterrupted time to properly use your dilator to help the vagina open and become flexible.

How to use the dilator:

Begin with the smallest sized dilator. Try to relax all of your muscles, especially in your vaginal area. A warm bath or shower can help you relax. Run warm water over the dilator to warm it up. Spread some water-based lubricant over the smallest end of the dilator (oil-based lubricant may dissolve the latex or plastic). Lie down and carefully place the smallest end of the smallest dilator into your vagina. If you want, you can use a dilator while you are in a warm bath. If the dilator does not slide into your vagina easily, glide the dilator only as far as it will go without pain. Then tense your vaginal muscles and release them. Slide the dilator a little further into your vagina and repeat the process of tensing and relaxing. If you can't move the dilator very far into the vagina, keep tensing and relaxing your muscles until you can gently move the dilator slowly into the vagina. Be careful not to force the dilator into your vagina. It may take several attempts or sessions before you can move it completely into your vagina. When the dilator is fully into your vagina (the base of the dilator will be near the outside of your vaginal opening), lie still and just try to relax for a few minutes. You may need to hold the dilator in your vagina with one hand as they have a tendency to slip out in the beginning. Carefully slide the dilator out of your vagina and then wash it with soap and thoroughly rinse it with water.

Once that step becomes comfortable, begin to practice this process every other day while increasing the time you leave in the dilator; try to work your way up to leaving the dilator in for at least 10 minutes. When that step becomes comfortable, try gently wiggling the dilator in your vagina and sliding it in and out. Remember to always use a lubricant. Continue this process until moving the smallest dilator around in your vagina is comfortable. Once this sized dilator becomes comfortable, it is time to move up to the next sized dilator and repeat the whole process until you are able to move up to the penis-sized dilator.

Discontinue using a dilator and consult your physician immediately if you experience sharp pain or bleeding after using a dilator.

DON'T FORGET TO BRING THE HUMOR

Ellen* had end-stage vaginal cancer and was hospitalized for removal of her vagina. Before her husband's visits, the nurses would make sure Ellen and the whole room smelled pleasant (vaginal cancer can be odorous) to keep up her self-esteem. When her vagina was removed, Ellen had to expand her new opening to allow for possible intercourse at a later time. As her nurse, I helped her by inserting a small dilator into the new opening and replacing it with increasingly larger dilators, as she grew ready. Intimacy was still important to Ellen and her husband, even with terminal cancer. One morning as I carried in the largest dilator, Ellen greeted me by joking with me about why I was there. Ellen's humor was infectious. From then on, I entered the room by telling her it was time for us to "get together." We were able to laugh together at a difficult situation.

Marsha Kooken, Oncology Nurse

Once you have begun to use a dilator, it is possible to involve your partner if you wish. When you are ready to become intimate, your partner can help you insert the dilator into your vagina. Choose a smaller-sized dilator than the one you are privately using on your own; otherwise, you will not enjoy this foreplay as it may cause pain. Your partner can help gently and seductively move the dilator into your vagina. If you prefer, your partner can instead insert a finger into your vagina during lovemaking until you are ready for his penis. Make sure your partner first puts lubrication on his finger. Again, it is important to relax your vaginal muscles, so you might try tensing them up and then relaxing them just before your partner inserts his finger. Your partner can increase the number of fingers as you become comfortable over time by practicing with your dilators. You can also have oral sex or attempt an orgasm by caressing each other until you are ready for intercourse. Just be careful not to insert anything into the vagina until you are ready.

When you have completed practicing with the largest dilator, you are probably ready for intercourse with your partner. Getting to this stage may take weeks or months, so be patient if your goal is to have intercourse. Even when you are ready for intercourse, you must both be very slow, gentle, and careful. Both of you need to lubricate first. Put a lot of lubrication in your vagina, outside your vagina, and on his penis. Try positioning yourself on top at first, as this is the easiest position to slide the penis into the vagina. Again, it is a good idea to squeeze your vaginal muscles and then relax them before inserting the penis into your vagina. (See Kegel exercises for a reminder if needed.) Go slow and steady. You may have to squeeze the muscles and relax a few times in order for the penis to completely enter your vagina. Remember to be gentle and careful with intercourse. You may be the only one who moves your hips during lovemaking the first few times. It might also help for you to continue to use dilators privately to keep your vaginal muscles relaxed and open.

A HUMMING, PLEASANT ROAD TO TRAVEL?
VIBRATORS

If you think you could never use a vibrator or that a vibrator is only for "that kind of girl," think again. In your circumstance, a vibrator is actually a medical device that can aid in your recovery from annoying or severe menopausal symptoms. Medical research has found that using a vibrator helps maintain the integrity of the vagina and reduces painful intercourse associated with symptoms of menopause.[1] If your beliefs or faith prevent you from masturbation, we respect that. But we also want to explain that using a vibrator to heal a dry, thinning, and narrowing vagina is like using a cane to walk until your leg heals.

When you are aroused and have an orgasm, blood flows to the tissues in your vagina and vulva, which causes moisture to build up (secrete) into your vagina. For a woman with a dry, tight, thin vagina, stimulation and sexual activity are important. Having an orgasm actually keeps the tissues in your vagina healthy.

That being said, your erogenous zones may have changed since you were treated for cancer. If your breasts are no longer there or are numb, they are not part of your sexual script. You won't be aroused when your partner touches your breasts or the place where your breasts used to be. You have to find new erogenous zones. A vibrator can help you explore your own body in private. It may also be easier to insert a vibrator covered with lubrication into a tight, dry vagina than a penis. This is especially true if you have sudden or aggravated menopausal symptoms

> *In your circumstance, a vibrator is actually a medical device that can aid in your recovery from annoying or severe menopausal symptoms.*

from cancer treatment. Perhaps your body appearance has changed or you are not yet emotionally ready to connect physically with your partner. You may just want some alone time to learn about what feels good, what doesn't, and what parts of your body are still in working order. Again, a vibrator can be your cane while you learn to walk again.

If you are single, using a vibrator is a great opportunity to explore yourself and soothe sexual frustrations that can build up after cancer treatment. You also need to figure out what feels good and what doesn't now so you'll be ready to tell a partner what you enjoy when you want to make love again.

Experimenting with self-stimulation after cancer may be a reassuring and helpful way to resume sex after cancer. While the topic of masturbation may still be taboo in parts of our society, try to think of a vibrator as what it is in your case: a medical treatment. Keeping your vagina stimulated and blood flowing to the surrounding tissue will actually help it heal. The Use It or Lose It theory at work again!

We spoke with leaders of various religious faiths about this subject, including one whose religion prohibits any kind of self-stimulation. The consensus was that cancer is a medical condition with real sexual medical consequences, and if using a vibrator or stimulating yourself to orgasm helps you heal, then it is a matter between you and God. We'll talk about this theory a little bit more in the chapter for husbands and partners too so that your partner will understand this concept. But again, using a vibrator is a personal decision and your choice alone. (See Chapter Seven for more detailed information on how to properly use the vibrator for self-stimulation.)

WHAT ARE OTHER OPTIONS?
COMPLEMENTARY AND ALTERNATIVE MEDICINES (CAMs)

First, it's important that you understand that CAMs do *not* have to be approved by the United States Food and Drug Administration (FDA). There are no long-term clinical trials to determine the side effects or safety of these products. These products do not contain package inserts as do FDA-approved medications, so you have very little medically-approved information when purchasing them. Another thing to consider is that there might be variations in the strength of each capsule contained within a single bottle.

Dr. Vibha Patel, a family practice physician in Fort Worth, Texas, says, "Natural doesn't mean safe. That's the biggest thing that I have to educate my patients about, explaining the safety issues of natural products." Always check with your doctor before trying any natural or herbal product. Herbs and other complementary therapies may interact poorly with your current prescription and nonprescription medications. Dr. Patel explains, "Your doctor may be hesitant to recommend complementary therapies. Find a physician who would be willing to talk with you about your questions and concerns regarding your complementary and alterative therapies."

Given that cautionary information, a botanical product called Zestra is available. Zestra is a blend of herbs that together act as a warming fluid to help lubricate and stimulate the clitoris. It is not clear exactly which herbs are in Zestra. It apparently works when it is gently massaged onto the clitoris and other parts of the vulva. Zestra can be used during foreplay, vaginal sex, manual stimulation, and masturbation. While it is safe to swallow Zestra, it's not flavored and not intended for use with oral sex. Zestra may help you have an orgasm because it brings blood flow to the area. We have heard from a few women that Zestra became too hot and unpleasant for them to continue to use (and remember that if burning is one of the problems you experience, Zestra may not be right for you.). You can obtain a sample of Zestra from your doctor or purchase Zestra online at web sites such as www.zestraforwomen.com or www.walgreens.com. If you are using condoms, use a polyurethane condom and not a latex condom with Zestra as it can damage latex condoms.

Many women try black cohosh, yams, or soy to reduce hot flashes and other symptoms of menopause. Not every "natural" product is safe for you after cancer. These products all contain "natural" estrogens that could be unsafe if you've had a hormone-sensitive cancer. Soy and herbal products such as black cohosh or products made with yams can convert into estrogen, although the jury is still out on the safety of using these products after cancer. Research is divided about the amount of soy or black cohosh you would have to take on a daily basis to increase your risk of recurrent cancer. Do not use a lubricant or other complementary therapy that contains natural phytoestrogens without first discussing it with your doctor.

Another herbal product on the market used to reduce painful intercourse is Avlimil Complete. Again, the FDA has not approved the safety of Avlimil Complete. It is a blend of herbs that includes soy and black cohosh, among others. It claims to reduce menopausal symptoms of hot flashes and mood swings, and possibly increase energy levels, physical comfort during sex, and libido, although these claims have not been substantiated by clinical research.

Another product some women have tried to reduce menopausal symptoms is DHEA (dehydroepiandrosterone). Dr. Vibha Patel would *not* recommend that a woman use DHEA after cancer treatment, however. DHEA is related to testosterone and estrogen. Do not take DHEA if you had a hormone-sensitive cancer. It is possible that DHEA can convert into testosterone and estrogen, which makes it unsafe after hormone-dependent cancers. It's a good idea to talk with your doctor about using DHEA before you try it, even if your cancer was not hormone-sensitive.

Also, remember that a natural hormone will not increase your sex drive; it may only help relieve menopausal symptoms, such as hot flashes or painful intercourse. Sitosterol is a natural estrogen that comes from soybean. It should be listed on the label of any product you plan to use, so read the label carefully before you try it. If you are unsure whether you can use a particular natural product to enhance your sex life, check with your doctor.

As Dr. Eshwar Kumar says, "Everything in moderation. The safety of using natural remedies such as soy or black cohosh is not yet fully understood. Quantify the risks: the amount you must take in order to increase your risks may be in the tons. Use a practical approach and discuss this issue with your doctor." Fortunately, if you decide the risks are too great, there are many other options that can relieve your menopausal symptoms after cancer treatment.

CAN I USE BIOIDENTICAL HORMONES?

Many women are confused about bioidentical hormones and wonder if they are "natural and safe" hormones. Hormones are hormones. A compound works the same way as the source that it comes from, whether it is from a plant or a synthetic material. So if the plant, like yams or soy, contains estrogen, the product you're using made from these plants will also contain estrogen. Using bioidentical hormones after having a hormone-sensitive cancer is just as risky as using older synthetic hormones. The difference between bioidentical hormones and older hormone therapies is simply the way the bioidentical hormones are processed and absorbed by your body. Your body might more easily absorb biodenticals because they are processed similarly to the way your body creates and processes hormones. However, this doesn't make them safer for you to use after cancer. If you want to try bioidentical hormones, talk with your doctor first; especially if your menopausal symptoms are severe or bothersome.

NON-HERBAL CAMs

We believe in the mind-body connection in healing. We've already talked about how the biggest sex organ in a woman's body is her mind. The connection between your mind and your physical desire for intimacy is real. So it goes for the healing of your whole body and mind after cancer. There are some complementary therapies available that may help you reduce stress, fatigue, and depression, which might allow you to spend more energy on your love life and increase your desire.

First, there is a great deal of information in print and on the Internet about alternative therapies. Proceed with caution. Second, it is important to run any kind of complementary therapy that you are thinking of trying past your doctor first, especially since you had cancer.

Eating a well-balanced diet, taking the right amount of the right vitamins (not mega doses), and getting enough sleep work together to enhance a healthy lifestyle. Adding gentle, moderate exercise, such as yoga, walking, or water aerobics may reduce stress, anxiety, and depression and actually give you more energy. More energy equals more willingness to think about intimacy.

> *"...I would have liked to be told about, when I was diagnosed...*
> *meditation, visualization. I never practiced it but I know*
> *it brings you tremendous inner peace and I would have liked*
> *to be steered to that approach in order to help me unwind, to*
> *remove that little distress I was feeling inside, all the fear I*
> *had, you know, really, to learn to relax..."*
>
> *Anonymous,*
> *(As quoted in <u>Nothing Fit Me: The Information</u>*
> *<u>and Support Needs of Canadian Young Women</u>*
> *<u>with Breast Cancer.</u> 2003 Final Report)*

Visualization therapies, such as guided imagery, and an active spiritual life may also improve your overall health.

Guided Imagery:

This is a way to relax using your imagination. It's based on the idea that your body and mind are connected. You use all of your senses: vision, hearing, feeling, smell, and taste. A common guided imagery experience is to imagine yourself lying on a warm beach. Try to hear the sounds of the ocean, feel the warmth of the sun and the sand, smell the ocean, and feel the sprays of the waves crashing into the beach. The body responds to this imagery by increasing blood flow through all of your tissues. It's a good example of the mind/body connection with complementary therapy. Some people say that practicing these visualizations, slowing down their breathing, relaxing, and enjoying this time has reduced pain and stress after cancer.

Prayer or Meditation:

Many studies have linked health to an active prayer or meditation life. In a recent study, researchers found that those who prayed even a few times a month had a better chance of staying healthy than those who didn't.[2] This is true for people who meditate without religious beliefs as well. When a person meditates, she clears all thoughts from her mind or she may concentrate or repeat a particular word or phrase. Meditation has been shown to lower blood pressure and decrease the risk of heart disease.[3] Adding prayer or meditation to your daily life just makes sense.

It's normal to be angry about having been diagnosed with cancer. Many of you may still be very angry at God. While it's normal, it's not necessarily healthy to hold on to this anger.

> *I was very angry at God. I had all of these friends who had nice lives. It didn't seem fair. It wasn't fair. I am still working on that.*
>
> *Mickey,*
> *(as quoted in The Breast Cancer*
> *Companion by Kathy LaTour)*

> *...that's the one part of your life that you're really mad at.*
> *Cancer survivor, Halifax, Nova Scotia, Canada*
> *(as quoted in Nothing Fit Me: The Information*
> *and Support Needs of Canadian Young Women*
> *with Breast Cancer, 2003 Final Report)*

If you can make peace with yourself, God, and your anger, you can move forward with your life. When you are ready, let it go. It's important not to let anger hold you back from living the full gift of life that lies in front of you, no matter how long you have. Releasing anger in your life will only free you from its burden...when you are ready. Remember, you are the one who is holding the anger, and you are the one who carries that weight. It can be heavy at times, and it is easier to let it go. You can write down two lists detailing the advantages and disadvantages of holding on to anger. You might be surprised at what you discover.

On the other hand, you may have been renewed or strengthened spiritually since cancer. In this case, you're probably already benefiting from the healing power of releasing anger and practicing prayer or meditation. You already know its positive influences.

I have often equated my experience with breast cancer to ten years of instant therapy sessions. In a flash we have been taken to the very core of our existence. Sometimes what we find there is not what we expect, and if our faith is something we wrap around us instead of inviting inside, we soon find ourselves on shaky ground...Song was another great release for me, and I sing songs while I drive, most of which I learned in church. These songs move me and help me feel the presence of the Lord. Some days when I am driving and feeling sorry for myself, a hymn will begin to get me out of myself and I look at the world outside the window and see the people who have so much less than I in terms of comfort and community. It never fails to get me back on track. As my daughter has gotten older, we have begun to sing in the car together. Whatever works on your spirit and soul is healing.

Kathy LaTour, Journalist, Cancer Survivor, and
Author of The Breast Cancer Companion

There are many complementary therapies available to reduce the stress in your life: art, music, pets, or even deep breathing exercises. For some women, massage therapy has helped. However, check with your doctor first if you have metastatic cancer as you may not be able to participate in massage therapy. The best advice is to find what works for you to reduce stress, anger, depression, and anxiety and run it past your doctor. Improving these issues will release more energy to participate in the important aspects of your life, including intimacy.

DEVELOPING TREATMENTS

It might help you to know that much is being done to investigate solutions for female sexual problems. New treatments are being developed, so ask your doctor regularly if there are any new treatments for your cancer-related menopausal symptoms or lost desire.

FACT OR FICTION?

*"You can use estrogen cream or topical estrogen when
you've had estrogen-positive cancer."*

FACT *AND* FICTION! The reality is that this decision is between you and your doctor. If your menopausal symptoms after cancer treatment are severe, your doctor may prescribe a local, low-dose estrogen cream. Your medical history and current symptoms will help you and your doctor decide what is safe for you.

---

[1] Billups KL (2002). The role of mechanical devices in treating female sexual dysfunction and enhancing the female sexual response. World Journal of Urology, 20(2): 137–141.

[2] Helm HM, Hay JC, et al. (2000). Does private religious activity prolong survival? A six-year follow-up study of 3,851 older adults. The Journals of Gerontology, Series A, Biological Sciences and Medical Sciences, 55(7): M400-5.

[3] Castillo-Richmond A, Schneider RH, et al. (2000). Effects of Stress Reduction on Carotid Atherosclerosis in Hypertensive African Americans. Stroke, 31(3): 568-73.

SIX

My Heart Hurts... Stolen Joy

How can I think of sex when such a life-changing event has occurred?

Paulette*, 44

You've learned about the physical changes that can occur after cancer treatment. Yet you might also be adjusting to significant psychological changes. Are these changes less important simply because they involve emotion? Absolutely not! You face a multitude of potential psychological challenges after cancer and its treatment. These challenges play a significant role in how you feel about intimacy, sex, and your relationships in general. All of your vital relationships may be affected, including:

1. Your relationship with yourself and how you perceive yourself
2. Your relationship with your intimate partner
3. Your relationships with extended family members, friends, and even the health professionals who provide ongoing care

You already know the importance of body image, self-esteem, and reducing stress in your life after cancer. These are very real problems that can significantly reduce your desire for intimacy, and not just sexual intercourse. Remember the mind-body connection. What happens in your physical body affects your mind, and what goes on in your mind affects your physical body. You are a complex, beautiful soul who is connected to powerful, necessary emotions.

PSYCHOLOGICAL CAUSES OF LOST DESIRE

More than likely you're trying to figure out who you are now, since cancer. You may be grieving for how your life used to be, before cancer. You may be grieving the loss of body parts or the loss of who you were before cancer. You may feel that your future will be more uncertain than you once believed it would be before your diagnosis. If you are a young woman, you may be concerned about whether or not having a child is possible, or grieving because you know it is no longer an option. The inability to bear children or the loss of the person you used to be are great losses that deserve some time to grieve. If you are dealing with sudden menopause symptoms or a lack of desire, you may be wondering if sex or intimacy means the same to you now.

There are a number of valid explanations for your unhappiness after cancer. Those of us who have had cancer know you can be:

- Genuinely saddened by the experience
- Traumatized by what you have experienced
- Actively mourning either past losses or future losses (for example, if you can no longer have a child)
- Depressed

Depression is common in people who have a chronic or traumatic illness. Depression frequently occurs along with conditions such as heart disease, diabetes, arthritis, and cancer. It can be triggered by the physical changes to your body caused by the disease, by medications used to treat the illness, or a psychological response to the disease.

> *What is wrong with me? I should be so happy that I am alive, but I am sad and depressed.*
>
> Patricia*, 49

In Chapter Two, we talked about the role of depression after cancer and its impact on your desire for an intimate love life. Depression affects every area of your health and functioning. Depression can make you feel lethargic and tired, which easily leads to a loss of sexual interest, among other things. It is a serious, chronic condition that needs treatment. If you think you are depressed, call your doctor or other health professional to schedule an appointment.

Dr. Vibha Patel says her patients are sometimes surprised to learn that depression is a real disease. "Depression is a medical condition based upon a collection of symptoms," says Dr. Patel. "It doesn't mean you're crazy." Several million Americans are diagnosed with depression every year, so you're not alone.

If you are unsure whether or not you have depression, take the following self-assessment to help you decide.[1]

DEPRESSION SELF-TEST

Check the boxes beside each statement if they apply to you:

☐ I feel sad, depressed, or am tearful much of the time.

☐ Most of the time, I am not interested in nor do I enjoy my work or other things that I used to take pleasure in, including friends, family, hobbies, activities, etc.

☐ I have recently been gaining or losing weight, and my appetite has changed. I am either eating too much or too little but have not been dieting.

☐ I have trouble sleeping, or I am sleeping too much.

☐ I often feel as if (a) I can hardly move, or (b) I am agitated or irritable.

☐ I feel tired or lack energy most of the time.

☐ I feel worthless or guilty nearly every day.

☐ I can't think or concentrate, or I have trouble making decisions, nearly every day.

☐ I frequently think of death or suicide.

If you have checked at least five boxes, and one of them is either the first or second item, it is possible that you are depressed. However, if you have these symptoms and someone you loved recently died, you may be experiencing grief and not depression. Even so, it is important to check with your doctor, a mental health professional (psychologist, licensed counselor, or psychiatrist), or a doctor in a hospital or clinic if you think you might be depressed. A self-help book cannot diagnose or treat your depression.

OTHER PSYCHOLOGICAL
CHALLENGES AFTER CANCER

We as a society are not comfortable discussing sexual issues. Period. Not with our lover, our close friends, and especially not our doctor. After surviving cancer or continuing to live with it, we may feel we shouldn't bother our doctors with issues of intimacy. We should just be satisfied with being alive, right?

Wrong. Let's say it together: **WRONG!**

We have a right to be fully informed about our sexual functioning. After cancer, we have a right to enjoy every aspect of our life, including sex and intimacy...we fought hard for this right during our battle with cancer.

Look in the mirror and say to yourself out loud, "I fought hard for my right to be fully alive, connected to myself and my lover, and to enjoy every part of my life, including intimacy with my partner."

Did you say it and mean it? We hope so. So let's get to the bottom of some of the other psychological reasons for decreased interest in intimacy and an active love life. What else impacts your desire besides depression?

DEMANDS OF EVERY DAY LIFE

Life is stressful, even without cancer. As women, we multitask and take care of everyone and everything. Do you run a home and manage to keep things functioning smoothly? Do you work outside the home, where demands for successful performance, the paycheck, and preserving health benefits keep you stressed and anxious? Do you have a partner or husband who needs your attention? Maybe you are a mom with small children who demand your time and attention. Maybe you have teenagers who challenge you in other ways. Take all of the normal demands in your life, and then add cancer and its treatment.

Add anxiety and the very real threat of death. Add to that the wondering if you will live to watch your children get old, travel to all those places you wanted to see with your mate, and do all that you wanted to do in this lifetime. Then there are the side effects of cancer treatments: fatigue, weight gain, or disfigurement. Combine all of these stressors together, and you wonder why you don't have any interest in sex? Did you think it was imagined or that something was wrong with you? If you answer "yes," then we urge you to think again. The mere fact that you are here, reading this book, and wondering about your love life is a testimony to your strength and courage. It is confirmation of your resolve, persistence, bravery, and your desire to live a full, treasured life. Give yourself a standing ovation...we are!

George was an old-fashioned man who thought housework was woman's work! But then he read that women who care for their families, make every meal, do all of the housework, and work outside the home are usually too tired for sex. George loved sex!

George took action. He cleaned the house like a mad man. He cooked the children's dinner, gave them baths, helped them with homework, and got them into bed before his wife came home from a long day of working. His wife was shocked when she entered the house and found a hot meal waiting and the whole house sparkling clean.

After telling her friends about the evening, one asked, "So how was the rest of your evening?" "Oh that was incredible too... Geoge was too tired..."
(Widely circulated urban legend and Internet joke)

It's not difficult to see why you are tired. Fatigue interferes with not only your ability to engage in sexual activity but also with your interest. During and after cancer treatment, your body is working hard to heal and make you well. Be kind to yourself. As we mentioned above, try to determine which responsibilities in your life could be handed over to others. Making time to nurture your love life, not just your sexual relationship, is vital.

SOLUTIONS TO COMMON PSYCHOLOGICAL INTIMACY PROBLEMS

You can start the psychological healing process by first acknowledging the physical and emotional losses and trauma that you have endured. This will help you process the pain and look beyond the devastation of cancer. Next, it is important to overcome negative thinking patterns, as discussed in Chapter Two. Work to improve your body image and learn to love yourself as you are now. Developing self-esteem skills will empower you to successfully change old, destructive thinking patterns. Another extremely important part of improving your need for intimacy is to communicate with your partner (see Chapter Eight for more information). Remember the vicious spiral of not having sex that we talked about earlier? Silence between you two about the quality of your love life is a killer. Start talking; you may be surprised that your beliefs about what your partner is thinking are wrong. You may both get a good laugh at the miscommunication. You may feel the reassurance that you need from your partner.

Try to keep an open mind about the way you feel sexual pleasure. Some women's vaginas will no longer allow penile penetration after cancer treatment. You may need to rewrite your former sexual script, the way you made love before cancer. There are so many other ways to enjoy your lover and for your lover to enjoy you both sexually and intimately. (See Chapter Seven for detailed information.)

Work with your mental health professional or doctor to better handle stress, depression, grief, and anxiety if you feel you need to. There is no shame in asking for this kind of help. You have carried a heavy burden, and learning new ways to cope with these challenges can only help you heal.

> **PROBLEM:** *No interest in intimacy or sex. You'd rather read a book or clean the toilet.*

> **SOLUTION:** *Read the right book and let someone else clean the toilet.*

If you think you'd rather read a book than become intimate with your partner, then read the right book! Watch the right movie, listen to the right music, and start feeling desirable again. Use sexual fantasy to get you thinking about intimacy and making love again.

> *If you think you'd rather read a book than become intimate with your partner, then read the right book!*

We know that for most men, this means making a trip to the video store's adult aisle. For women, it is more likely that a romantic book, movie, or song will make you feel sensuous or pique your interest in intimacy. Think about how good it would feel to be touched, cuddled, stroked, kissed, or just lie naked next to your lover. You have to ignite that part of your mind again, and the spark that lights the fire might just be a good "chick flick."

When you do become aroused or even remotely curious about intimacy again, eliminate external distractions so you can concentrate on each other. Make the atmosphere and environment sensual. Light candles, dim the lights, play soft or sexy music, have a glass of wine if you are able, and basically set the stage for this new act. Remember that men need a time and place to have sex. Women need a setting, an atmosphere, and emotional foreplay. Removing distractions will allow you to focus on you and your lover.

As women, we have a tendency to think about many things at once. We can lie there physically participating in sex but also be thinking about the dishes in the sink, the kids' school projects, and what we need from the grocery store. We cannot stress the importance of removing all distractions, even if you do not plan on having sexual intercourse. Turning off the TV to talk together can be a very romantic, intimate experience. Set the stage for the return of your love life. Start thinking about it again and what you want from your love life and your lover now. Start rewriting your sexual script.

> **PROBLEM: Grief, depression, anger, and anxiety prevent a return to intimacy.**

> **SOLUTION: Identify the problem(s), work through your feelings, and seek professional psychological help when needed.**

Grief is a normal response to a significant loss or change in your life. After cancer, you may experience one or more of the following:

- Physical loss, such as the loss of a breast or ovaries.
- An altered lifestyle; you can no longer participate in activities you used to enjoy.
- Loss of your identity, asking who am I now?
- Loss or shift of a significant relationship.

You may feel sorrow, sadness, emptiness, or heartache. You may wonder how long these emotions will last. When does grief become a problem?

Generally, there is no time limit on grief. It takes however long it takes, and each person moves through grief at a different speed. You may think you are fine one minute, and the next you feel the heartache again. This sequence can go on for weeks, months, or even years. Maybe the best rule of thumb for deciding whether grief has become a problem is to ask yourself, "Is grief interfering with my ability to live my life or to move forward with my life?" If the answer is, "Yes," then it may be time to seek care from a qualified mental health professional (such as a psychologist, counselor, or psychiatrist) so that you can move forward with your life.

Grief can affect you physically, emotionally, and socially. Typical symptoms of grief include:

- A heavy chest or tight throat
- An empty feeling
- Loss of appetite
- Feelings that alternate between guilt and anger
- Restlessness, difficulty concentrating
- Difficulty sleeping, fatigue
- Increased or unexpected crying;
- Headaches, dry mouth, stomach aches
- A feeling that the loss is not real
- Excessive worry or feelings of being vulnerable
- Increased concern for other family members

Grief often occurs along with feeling anxious, guilty, depressed, or worried. You may withdraw from your family and friends. Some women want to stay in bed and not get out. Or some women continue with all the normal activities but feel like "zombies" and are just going through the motions, feeling numb. Again, you may find yourself questioning your faith or spiritual beliefs at this time.

Grief can roll over you like a "sneaker wave" from the ocean; it sneaks up behind you and catches you when you're not looking. You will be fine one minute, but the next, you're in tears. When first grieving a loss, you can become tearful at the drop of a hat; the waves of grief are high and close together. As the grief process continues, the waves still seem high but appear further apart... little periods of "normal" living sprinkled

> *Grieving stresses your body and weakens your immune system.*

with overwhelming pain. As time goes on and you work through grief, the waves get smaller and further apart. However, just when you think the waves have subsided, you are drenched again. Grief never completely disappears, but over time, grief does appear far less frequently.

Physicians disagree on whether to treat grief with medications. If you have extreme difficulty sleeping, or coping with your daily life, your doctor may prescribe a mild, short-term sedative to help you sleep. Most doctors agree, however, that prescribing medications while you are grieving only masks the pain and doesn't allow you to move through the pain past grief. You will have to process the grief sooner or later. You may be able to mask the pain for a while, but realize you will have to deal with it eventually. Unresolved grief causes all sorts of problems.

Grieving stresses your body and weakens your immune system. A weakened immune system makes you susceptible to viruses, such as colds, or other illnesses. You might feel body aches or worsen an existing condition when grieving. Grief counseling can help you work through the grief. Your counselor can teach you about the grieving process and what you can expect as you move through it. Grief counseling can also be a safe place to express pent up feelings, or to work through those feelings.

A grief counselor can also help you decide your new identity after cancer. Sometimes, we need help answering the question, "Who am I now?"

Dr. William Worden, a clinical psychologist, talked about the four tasks of grief.[2] We've re-worked these tasks to reflect losses from cancer and its treatment.

1. Acknowledge the reality of your loss. Realize that you have lost something tangible, whether it is a sense of invulnerability, a breast, the ability to have children, or your innocence about life and death.
2. Feel the pain of grief. Yes, grieve...don't avoid it. Think of grief like a circle. Inside the circle is the pain. The quickest way to get to the other side of the circle is to go through it, not around it. The pain has to be processed sooner or later. You can grow through it. It will eventually get easier.
3. Adjust to a new, changed environment where you recognize your losses. You are different now. Acknowledge that you've lost a breast, or a uterus, or a vagina as a result of cancer. Work on coping with a breast that has no feeling, or the inability to have children, or a change in the way you are intimate with someone else.
4. Change the relationship you had with what you lost. Bid goodbye to the old you and embrace the new person in order to move forward with your life. It may not have been by choice, but you are a new person. Get to know this new person, care for her, support her, have a conversation with this new "you" and continue growing as a person.

Other things you can do while you are working through grief:

•   Eat regularly and eat well, even if it means eating small snacks throughout the day until you become hungry enough to eat a meal again.

- Try to stick to a schedule, such as going to bed and waking around the same time each day and sleeping nearly the same number of hours each night. Participate in your normal daily activities as best as you can. Keeping a schedule can bring "normal" back into your life even though you don't yet feel normal.
- Try to get gentle exercise every day. Just as with depression, some form of exercise may help reduce feelings of anxiety, grief, and loss. Take a walk, do yoga, or work in your garden.
- Acknowledge your pain and grief. Be kind to yourself. Surround yourself with a good support system, and if you are a spiritual person, practice your faith.

It is common to ponder the "if only's" during grief. "If only I hadn't taken hormone therapy..." or "If only I'd gone for a mammogram earlier..." We set unreasonably high standards for ourselves. When we don't move the ball forward but continue to focus on the "what ifs" of what we think we did or didn't do, we only end up feeling worse. This is not a good solution to moving through grief.

It can take a long time to move through the process of grief. However, if you think you are "stuck" in grieving, seek help. Grief can usually be treated with time and loving support from family, friends, or a counselor. A grief counselor can help you move through the pain and back into your life. Your love life and relationships with yourself and others will obviously improve once you have dealt with grief after cancer.

DEPRESSION, ANGER, ANXIETY

I thought I was doing well, taking my children to school, and doing daily activities. Then, out of the blue, I would start to cry, or felt panicked for no reason. I didn't feel this way all of the time, but I also didn't feel like my old self either. I didn't smile much and I can't remember the last time I laughed out loud.

Barbara*, 38

Left untreated, grief can lead to problems with anxiety, unresolved anger, and depression. Your relationship and intimacy issues will remain on the bottom of your list of importance as you deal with these very real emotions and medical conditions. If you took the self-assessment and think you may have depression, talk with a mental health professional or your doctor. Generally, counseling or a combination of medications and counseling are the preferred treatment for depression, even after cancer. Just because you take medications for depression doesn't mean that you are weak, and it also doesn't mean that you will have to take these medications for the rest of your life. Your body may need temporary help producing a chemical that helps regulate mood, such as serotonin, and there is nothing wrong with that. You would not think less of a person who takes insulin for diabetes, so don't be hard on yourself if you need depression medication for a while.

Try to work through the life issues that lead to depression. Medications should not be used as a quick fix for depression or for grief. Medications can be helpful, however, especially for depression that is linked to a decrease of certain brain chemicals that regulate mood. Once your body begins producing the proper chemicals again, and once you have learned helpful coping skills to deal with stress, grief, and loss after cancer, you may not need medications.

It is important that you talk with a qualified counselor and not merely take medications to treat depression or anxiety. Group therapy might also help. Gilda's Club (www.gildasclub.org) is an example of an organization that offers group therapy and helps many women touched by cancer. You can talk with other women in a similar situation and learn ways to express yourself in a supportive atmosphere.

> *PROBLEM: Body image, self-esteem, undesirable feelings after cancer.*
>
> *SOLUTION: Re-read Chapter Two, work on recognizing and acknowledging your value, and pay attention to how you look and feel.*

You've read about the importance of body image, self-esteem, and moving away from negative thinking about yourself in Chapter Two. You know how important it is to remember that as a woman, you are a powerful force of nature with or without your breasts or reproductive organs. You are still you...a former schoolgirl, teenager, daughter, wife, mother, grandmother, or lover...still a phenomenal woman!

Are you paying attention to how you look and feel? Are you dressing the way you dressed when you felt beautiful and attractive before cancer? Are you paying attention to your physical appearance, no matter how changed you are now? Do you wear your favorite jewelry? How about a little make up if you wore it before cancer? Do you dab perfume behind your earlobes, on your wrists, or where your cleavage once appeared? Do you dance and hum to your favorite song? Do you laugh at the jokes only women really "get"? Do you wear softness and strength on both the inside and outside? Do you feel like a woman?

Yes, you need to start healing from the inside out, but sometimes feeling good about yourself on the outside helps with the inside. Looking feminine (or however you feel desirable) on the outside may help with how you feel on the inside. It may also help you feel attractive. Think back to how you groomed or primped when you first began dating your lover. Did you pay a little more attention to your appearance, checking in the mirror again and again before your date arrived? Look, we're not trying to set the women's movement back a hundred years. Instead, we're trying to remind you how you paid attention to yourself, your looks, and the way you felt about yourself when you first began dating your partner. Go back to that place, both in your mind and outwardly, and you can begin again to rebuild the intimacy, attraction, and desire you had for each other when it all began. You get to fall in love all over again!

> **PROBLEM: Husband or partner no longer shows interest in intimacy or sex.**

> **SOLUTION: Communicate, communicate, communicate!**

Communication is one of the most significant components in healing intimacy and sexual problems in your relationship. A lack of communication is death to any relationship, especially to an intimate one. It is a passion killer in a marriage, a partnership, and especially to a romantic connection between the two of you. All too often, you believe your partner is thinking, feeling, or responding in a way he is not. You

> *A lack of communication is death to any relationship, especially to an intimate one.* ❖

project your feelings of inadequacy or unattractiveness onto your partner's thinking. He may very well be worried about your response to his pursuing intimacy with you again after cancer. He may simply be afraid. But as we mentioned earlier, when neither of you discusses these silences between you, the spiral of wrong thinking, no sex or intimacy, and hurt feelings begins its ugly and destructive passage. We discuss communications issues and solutions in more depth in Chapter Eight.

> *Before cancer, we had a fairly active sex life and definitely were close to one another emotionally. After my cancer treatment, my husband didn't approach me or even touch me, even though he was very attentive to my physical needs during treatment. Finally I couldn't stand it any longer. I tearfully cried out, "Why don't you touch me anymore? Why don't you want sex anymore? Am I that repulsive to you now?" My even-tempered husband quietly responded, "Of course I am attracted to you, but it is difficult to make love to an invalid. I'm afraid of hurting you." What I didn't understand was that my husband now thought of me as a sick person, an invalid, someone who needed care but not caressing. Once I was able to assure him I was well enough to be held and loved, we resumed our sex life, and it has been wonderful.*
>
> *Anna*, 51*

Remember that women and men communicate differently. When a woman has a burden, she releases it to her trusted girlfriends, who listen quietly, make her a cup of tea, and hug her while she cries. A man wants to fix it. When he can't fix it, he becomes frustrated and angry. Then he avoids what he cannot conquer. This is a little simplistic but overall, true. Your husband or partner may be avoiding you sexually because he is afraid or frustrated that he cannot fix what ails you.

You can help by working through any negative emotions you are feeling: depression, grief, anger, or anxiety. When you feel less sexual due to these emotions, as well as other psychological issues brought on by cancer, you just might be sending unspoken signals to your lover that sex and intimacy are out of the question. He may be responding to those signals by retreating, not rejecting you.

SOLUTIONS CONTINUE...

The problems mentioned above are commonly experienced by women after cancer and its treatment. The solutions offered work for many women, although you may need to individualize each solution for your specific situation. Should you find that you still have difficulties after trying the suggested solutions, remember there are many health professionals available to help you through each and every one of the problems you face since treatment, whether they are physical or psychological. You are worth the effort it might take to resume an active love life.

NORMAL AGING VERSUS CANCER SYMPTOMS

Are your sexual symptoms a result of cancer and its treatment, or is it possible they are a result of normal aging? When a traumatic event like cancer enters our life, we have a frame of reference for what has occurred *before* the event and *after* the event. We have a tendency to attribute all aches, pains, depression, loss of sex drive, and any other new symptom we have *after* the illness to that illness or event. Some women say, "Look what cancer has done to me," when in fact, it is simply a result of normal aging.

Be careful not to blame cancer for everything.

Yes, cancer and its treatment can cause significant changes to our bodies, with symptoms that linger for weeks, months, years, or even for the rest of our lives. However, normal aging can also cause similar symptoms. How do you tell the difference, and is it important to know the source of the symptoms?

If you are a woman between the ages of 39 and 51, it's possible you might already be experiencing some of the symptoms of perimenopause or menopause. Perimenopause means "around menopause" and spans the 2 to 8 years before menopause when hormone levels begin to change. Menopause occurs 12 months after your last menstrual period. Symptoms of perimenopause and menopause can include itching, dry vagina, loss of interest in sex, trouble sleeping, mood swings, irritability, depression, problems concentrating or recalling words, hot flashes, night sweats, headaches, and trouble becoming sexually aroused, which can lead to painful intercourse. During perimenopause, you'll notice changes in your menstrual cycles, such as a heavier or lighter than normal bleeding and your cycles become shorter or longer. No treatment is usually needed for menopause. Some women who have not had cancer or a hormone-sensitive cancer try hormone therapy or herbal therapies, such as black cohosh or soy, under medical supervision to relieve perimenopausal symptoms. This may not be an option for you after cancer, especially if you had a hormone-sensitive cancer, so be sure to check with your doctor first. Other effective non-medical treatments for symptoms of menopause are good nutrition, rest, exercise, and using relaxation techniques, such as deep breathing exercises.

Perimenopause and menopause are a normal part of aging. However, the severity of menopausal symptoms can be considerably worsened by cancer treatment. Cancer treatment can also cause a younger woman to go into early menopause. It's possible that the flare up of menopausal symptoms will calm down once cancer treatment has stopped.

Fatigue is another common symptom in women with busy lives. You are pulled in several different directions when caring for a family or even when you are single and work full time. Busy lives lead to fatigue, and fatigue has a way of eliminating desire. Some of us just don't want to be bothered with sex, although most of us still enjoy the intimacy of our loving relationship. Why would we want to add one more thing to our already overflowing list of "Things I have to do." As we mentioned earlier, it might be time to re-evaluate your long list of obligations, remove those you can, and hopefully eliminate some of that fatigue that keeps you from wanting to make love.

A woman was sitting at a bar enjoying an after work cocktail with her girlfriends when an exceptionally tall, handsome, extremely sexy middle-aged man entered. He was so striking that the woman could not take her eyes off him.

The young-at-heart man noticed her overly attentive stare and walked directly toward her (as all men will). Before she could offer her apologies for so rudely staring, he leaned over and whispered to her, "I'll do anything, absolutely anything, that you want me to do, no matter how kinky, for $20...on one condition." (There are always conditions.)

Flabbergasted, the woman asked what the condition was.

Then he replied, "You have to tell me what you want me to do in just three words." (Controlling, eh?)

The woman considered his proposition for a moment, and then slowly removed a $20 bill from her purse, which she pressed into the man's hand along with her address. She looked deep into his eyes, and meaningfully said....

"Clean my house."

      (Widespread urban legend and Internet joke)

If you are a younger woman with menopausal symptoms since cancer treatment, your treatment likely caused your symptoms. Your symptoms may improve once treatment is over and hormonal imbalances are resolved. Stress, depression, or grief may also contribute to your lost sex drive. It is possible, then, that your lack of interest in sex and intimacy will not fully return even when your other physical symptoms, such as dry, tight vagina, improve. It's important to keep talking with your doctor about all of your symptoms until you are physically and emotionally well again, and this includes the return of your sex drive.

You and your doctor may not always be able to tell which symptoms are a direct result of cancer treatment and which are related to normal aging. The most important thing is to keep talking with your doctor, finding the best solutions to your physical and emotional issues, and living your life, including your sex life, to the fullest.

SEX AND INFERTILITY

Now that I can't conceive a baby since chemo made me sterile,
I'm not so sure if sex even matters anymore.

Kate*, 34

For the woman still wanting biological children, cancer and its treatment can shatter all of your hopes and dreams. Hopefully, your doctor talked at length with you about the consequences of certain cancer treatments before you were treated. Even so, the loss of the dream for future biological children is immeasurable for some...the grief unbearable. We honor and acknowledge your grief. We know it will take time for you to move through it. But we hope you do, and that you are able to connect with your partner in this grief, so the two of you can share it together, move through it together, and become intimately closer than ever.

There are many wonderful books written about infertility after cancer. One book we recommend is entitled <u>Sexuality and Fertility After Cancer</u>, by Leslie R. Schover, Ph.D.[3] In it, she spends time discussing the pain of infertility after cancer and options for preserving your egg and preventing infertility before cancer treatment begins. For our purpose, we are writing for those women who have already received cancer treatment, are now infertile, and wonder about the significance of sex and intimacy in their lives.

While acknowledging your loss, the bottom line is that intimacy and an active sex life still matter, whether or not you can bear children. Lovemaking is part of your existence and function as a human being. Intimacy is about being loved, valued, treasured, and acknowledged. We all need love. We may not all need intercourse, but we all need affection, kindness, and to know that our existence matters. We were created for this purpose...to love and be loved.

But you might ask, "Where does sex fit in now? It doesn't mean the same to me anymore." Again, it is a matter of rewriting your sexual script. You may have equated sex with pregnancy before cancer. Now you can equate it with sheer pleasure, a time to focus on your needs and those of your lover. If you were sexually reserved before, maybe it's time to buy some sex toys. If you were more "wild" before cancer, maybe it's time to focus on the quieter, intimate aspect of lovemaking...the tender, soft communication of it all.

QUESTIONS FOR YOUR DOCTOR

If you are uncomfortable asking your doctor questions about intimacy, we can get you started. Remember, it's important to talk with the doctor you feel most comfortable with, regardless of whether she is your gynecologist, oncologist, or primary care provider. If he or she is unable to answer the questions you have about your sex life, then ask your doctor to recommend someone who can.

NEVER IN THE SAME BREATH: SEX AND CANCER

Doctors don't often bring up sexual issues when treating cancer. In fact, most doctors don't discuss it – sex is all about life, and cancer is...well, not. One cancer survivor brought up her sexual symptoms repeatedly with her doctor only to be patted on the head and told, "You have so much on your plate right now, why would you worry about that?" Another survivor tells us that when she finally did get the courage to bring up sexual issues with her doctor, he grew red in the face, obviously embarrassed, and simply stared at his shoes until she gathered her things and left. What we must remember is that doctors are human. They are also not trained to discuss sexual problems with their patients—it's embarrassing to them sometimes too. And, to be fair, medical students don't usually go into oncology training because they want to talk about sex. That just needs to be something they learn along the way, or we hope they do.

You may see your oncologist more than any other doctor right now, and you can always start there. Or, if you prefer, ask your oncology nurse if your oncologist is the right person to talk with about some intimacy issues you're having since treatment. The nurse may be able to help you avoid an embarrassing conversation if the oncologist is not going to be comfortable with that discussion, and also help you find the right doctor. Another appropriate doctor to see about intimate matters is your OB/GYN. He or she is well educated in menopause and its symptoms and can work with your oncologist to provide the safest treatment for menopausal symptoms after cancer. You may prefer to speak with your primary care doctor, and that is appropriate too.

QUESTIONS TO HELP YOU GET THE CONVERSATION STARTED

1. How is my cancer treatment likely to affect my love life? How will the medications affect my love life?

2.   I'm concerned about side effects of treatment that involve intimacy issues. Are you the right doctor to talk with about these issues? If not, could you give me the name of a doctor who could help me with these issues?

3.   Can we talk about some severe menopausal symptoms I'm having? This is ruining my love life. What do you recommend?

4.   Can you recommend a good gynecologist or primary care provider who can help me with some symptoms that have interfered with my love life since I've been treated for cancer?

5.   Is there anything I can do about the side effects of treatment that interfere with my marital relationship?

6.   I'm having the side effects you warned me about that would cause symptoms of menopause. Can you help me with those symptoms or is there another doctor I should see?

7.   I'm having symptoms of menopause since treatment. Can you treat these symptoms or send me to another doctor?

8.   What are the long-term side effects after treatment? (E.g., what menopausal symptoms can I expect and are there remedies?)

9.   What can my husband expect from my long-term side effects? (Some couples are okay to discuss this topic together, and some are not. Interestingly, many women start the conversation for men who have lost potency due to cancer.)

10. If you are too shy to ask the questions, see if your partner will ask them for you.

Dr. Eshwar Kumar says, "A woman can speak to her family doctor if the oncologist is embarrassed to talk about this subject. She can ask for a recommendation or simply go back to her family doctor for the recommendation." Dr. Kumar adds, "Do not be embarrassed to ask the question. Quality of life is a huge issue and something as professionals we tended not to recognize before, and this needs to be corrected. If a physician is uncomfortable discussing sex, he or she can just say, 'I don't know enough about this subject but can refer you to someone who will.'"

We know that some of you have already attempted to talk with a doctor about the very personal issues you face since cancer treatment, only to have that doctor be more embarrassed about the conversation than you. Please don't let this prevent you from asking another, qualified doctor about the intimacy issues you face. There is a doctor out there who can help you. It might take a few tries to find him or her. We have talked to many doctors about this topic. Some admit to being embarrassed, but they all said they were prepared to talk about it. If you are unfortunate and have come across the one doctor who doesn't want to discuss it, ask for a referral to someone else who will. Most importantly, know this: you are responding very normally to a very abnormal situation.

Dr. Kumar explains, "From a professional perspective, I used to think these were issues for the younger generation. They are not. Age should not be a barrier for women asking these questions. Quality of life is very important at any age, not just for the young. Physicians and health professionals need to find out from their colleagues about these types of resources. We need to find out what and who is out there to help and to make the appropriate referrals." We couldn't agree with you more, Dr. Kumar.

FACT OR FICTION?

'Once you are treated for cancer, you are no longer fertile."

FICTION! Definitely not true! Many women are able to give birth after cancer treatment. Talk with your doctor about your options for having biological children before and after you are treated for cancer.

[1] American Psychiatric Association (2000). Depressive disorders. In Diagnostic and Statistical Manual of Mental Disorders, 4th ed., text rev., pp. 349–381. Washington, DC: American Psychiatric Association.

[2] Worden JW (2002). Grief Counseling and Grief Therapy: A Handbook for the Mental Health Practitioner, 3rd ed. New York: Springer Publishing Company, Inc.

[3] Schover LR (1997). Sexuality and Fertility After Cancer, pp. 157-186. New York: John Wiley & Sons, Inc. Reprinted with permission of John Wiley & Sons, Inc.

SEVEN

Bring Back that Loving Feeling

Sex is an emotion in motion...
When I'm good, I'm very good. But when I'm bad, I'm
better...

Mae West

We don't always know what we want from our love life, even without the intrusion of cancer. We have different needs and desires, along with various constraints, throughout the different stages of our lives. You may be wondering what you want or need sexually after cancer treatment. Perhaps you do not want sexual intercourse, but would like to improve the closeness or intimacy in your relationship. Now is the time to explore your options. It's time to rewrite or strengthen your "sexual script" or the way you love and express your sexual feelings. If your body has changed either through surgery or treatment for cancer, your erogenous zones have likely changed too. Seeking new ways to find pleasure can be a great adventure, both for you and your lover.

As you know, intimacy begins in a woman's mind. Are you thinking about love and romance again? Have thoughts of being held or sharing tender moments with your lover started to cross your mind? Light the candles, dim the lights, turn on the music, and set the proper mood. When you are ready, you can revive those old feelings, both emotionally and physically, that connect you with your lover. You might wonder how to begin again when you've had that imaginary sex neuron disconnected. All it takes is that one little spark to light the fire.

THURSDAY DINNER DATES

Diana Leitch, R.N. R.M.T., is an intimacy and sexuality counselor. She compares sex after cancer to a Thursday evening dinner date. You've worked all day, you're tired and just want read a good book or watch TV. But no, you have to go to a friend's house, which means you need to look nice, smell nice, and actually get into your car and leave the house again. Your energy level is zapped. However, because you committed to going earlier, you must show up. Grudgingly, you take off your comfortable sweatpants, shower again, fix your hair, "moisturize" (more on this later), put on your party dress, and out the door you go, grumbling all the way. You fake warm "Hello's" to your dinner party friends, find a comfortable chair, and grit your teeth for the duration. Then something happens. You're laughing with a friend you haven't talked with for awhile. You're really interested in what he is telling you about his own life. The food is actually quite good, and you take a second helping. You begin to feel a little energy, find that you are talkative, and suddenly realize that you genuinely enjoy being around these people. You look up at the clock; it is late. You're having a great time, are wide awake, laughing more than you've laughed in a long while, and you really don't want to leave the party. You're truly glad you went.

Renewing your love life after cancer can be like a Thursday dinner date. Getting off the couch and out of your sweatpants may be a struggle, but once there, you might really enjoy the party. Like Diana says,

*Sometimes you are looking to have a positive relationship with someone you care for, and I don't mean casual sex. Intimacy isn't casual; you have to nurture and feed intimacy in order for it to grow. Sometimes before bed, you might jump into the tub, keep on a little makeup, and wear a nightie that makes you feel pretty, whether or not it has one or two flat sides where your breasts used to be. You look pretty for **you**, not your lover, because it makes **you** feel good! It's worth the effort to feel good about how you look — we dress for ourselves! Sometimes, intimacy and sex are worth giving that extra little effort, like going to the Thursday night party. Sex may not be the prime driving force in your life, but when you make the effort for yourself (and don't do it just to please him but do it to please you), you can overcome the little bump in the road.*

NEW BEGINNINGS...JUST LIKE OLD TIMES
Your Sexual Script

What is a sexual script? It is the very personal choice of how you express intimacy and love. It has a beginning, middle, and an end. Your sexual script is the how, what, when, where, and why of your intimate and sexual relationship. For example, how do you transition from a nonsexual situation to a sexual one? In the beginning, do you wear sexy lingerie or drink a glass of wine? Do you have a set pattern, such as always making love on a Saturday night? What usually occurs before you become intimate; for instance, does your partner become playful with you by patting your bottom or pinching a breast? How do you respond? As you move to the middle of the script, who does what? For instance, who usually initiates lovemaking? How do you or your partner know the other is interested? Where do you usually make love? How do you set the mood? Does your sexual script end with intercourse and orgasms, or do you have another way of expressing yourselves sexually? Your unique sexual script is how you enjoy your intimate relationship. After cancer, that script might change.

For example, if your husband used to pinch your breasts to attract your attention, but now your breasts are numb or absent, he'll have to find another approach.

Men and women often need to reconcile their sexual scripts. In general, women prefer seduction, romance, and lingering foreplay. We usually want the lights out and like sex at night. Men typically want the lights on, spontaneity, visual stimulation, variety, and sex in the morning. Men want to see, women want to hear, "I love you." During foreplay, women are more likely to be "spectators" in that we notice the things around us, such as our sagging breasts or large stomachs. Men are more fully engaged in merely making love, not noticing what is going on around them or what a woman thinks are her physical faults. Women are more easily distracted during lovemaking by children or noises downstairs, whereas men tend to be much more focused.

Your spouse or partner may be a "breast" or a "butt" guy. One of you probably initiated sex more often, and you both followed a pattern when making love. For example, you may have signaled your desire to launch into lovemaking by turning a peck on the cheek into passionate kisses. After cancer, you might try to avoid the "launch sequence" for fear of having sex before you're ready. Your launch sequence might also have changed since treatment. What felt good before may now be uncomfortable or even painful. Many women must rewrite their sexual scripts after treatment. If you have a missing breast or now have an ostomy bag, the sexual script must change. Deciding the when, why, how, where, and what of your sexual and intimate life after cancer treatment is your decision to make. The first step is to simply begin thinking about it again, and decide what *you* now want from this part of your life.

> *Sexuality is the core of our being. It is what got us here in the first place. Sex is a huge part of our lives. It underscores the relationship we're in...a sexual script is individual. It's very personal, and has to do with our upbringing and the acceptance of our body more than it does with our age.*
>
> *Diana Leitch*

What was dating your partner like? Were you great kissers? If so, this is a wonderful place to begin again! Kissing can be erotic and bring you emotionally closer together. Did you like the way you looked then? If so, now is the time to return to appreciating who you are, just as you are. Do what makes you feel good about yourself. Pamper yourself. Remember what it was like to get ready for a date? Spending time picking out what you'd wear, putting on make up if you wore it, and making sure your breath was fresh. It's not about looking good for your partner; it is about feeling good about yourself. Go on a date with your partner again; spark the romance between you. Remember that for women, foreplay begins in our minds.

You might want to avoid intercourse after treatment because you are worried about or have already experienced pain during sexual contact. It's possible you're not sure what you want from your sexual relationship now. We're going to give you some ideas for writing a new sexual script. You get to decide how to write a new sexual script. The how, what, when, where, and why of making love is up to you. At some point, you may want to involve your partner's wishes too, but first, you get to decide what it is you need from your love life after cancer.

It is also important to note that not all sexual problems after treatment are related to cancer. Some sexual problems are due to not having learned about sex properly or if we were left guessing about sexual education. How did you find out about the facts of life? This can influence the way you respond to sex. Also, if you were taught that sex was "wrong," you may already be uncomfortable with sex, even if your discomfort is subconscious. Becoming properly sexually educated, learning about your body and how it functions, can help reduce anxiety around sex. Some women may have a history of abuse or other sexual issues that causes them anxiety. As Diana Leitch says, "The hooves you hear coming toward you may not be zebras but just ordinary horses." In other words, your sexual issues may not be cancer-related, especially if you have a history of abuse. If you think your current sexual concerns could be caused by something other than cancer treatment, a qualified sex therapist or mental health counselor with training in sexual abuse can help you work through these issues.

HOW DO I SET THE MOOD WITH AN OSTOMY BAG?

Your issue may not be a missing breast, but the addition of a medical device such as an ostomy bag. It's not something you can simply remove and replace after sex. It is, however, something you can hide or make secure so that you feel free to express yourself sexually. Oncology nurse Marsha Kooken suggests the following helpful hints for setting the mood when you have an ostomy bag.

1. Spontaneity might not be an option for a while. Plan your rendezvous; it will still be worth the effort. Give yourself a little time before your partner arrives to prepare yourself.

2. Set the mood the usual way: candles, soft music, and whatever else is normal for the two of you. One extra step, make sure the room smells nice. You have to spend a little more time controlling odor issues with an ostomy bag.

3. You probably don't want to undress in front of your partner. Seeing the contents of the bag can be a romantic turnoff. You can wear a bag cover to hide the contents.

4. Empty the bag just before you meet your partner. Do not open the bag anywhere but in the bathroom.

5. Use soap and water to clean the bag thoroughly. You'll want to make sure the bag is clean and free of gas. You probably don't want any "sound effects" while making love.

6. Lay a towel by the bed in case you spring a leak.

7. You may want to wear specially made lingerie that contains a pouch to hold and conceal your bag. The pouch keeps the bag secure so you don't have to worry about it detaching during sex. (See Chapter Two for more information on where to purchase lingerie.)

8. Remember that wild sex is not an option if your body is still fragile from cancer treatment. Go with gentle, easy lovemaking. You may want to position yourself on top of your lover for easier entry into the vagina.

This scheduled tryst and knowing how to properly prepare for your intimate encounter is lovely if you are ready to resume your sex life after cancer. However, if you wonder how to begin the romance again, we have a few suggestions to help you get started.

AND NOW...LET US BEGIN AGAIN!

A young man and his wife decided to save their marriage with counseling. When they arrived at the counselor's office, he asked, "What seems to be the problem?"

Immediately, the husband held his long face downward and said nothing. On the other hand, the wife began talking rapidly, describing all the wrongs within their marriage.

After listening to the wife, the counselor went over to her, picked her up by her shoulders, kissed her passionately for several minutes, and sat her back down.

The wife was speechless. The husband stared in disbelief at what had just happened. The counselor spoke to the husband, "Your wife NEEDS that at least twice a week!"

136   *Intimacy After Cancer: A Woman's Guide*

The husband scratched his head and replied, "Okay, I can have her here on Tuesdays and Thursdays."

(Widely spread urban legend and Internet joke)

All joking aside, sometimes you have to try new ways to figure out what feels good, especially if your body is altered by cancer treatment. Your "feel good zones" might have changed, and you may need to explore your body to find out what works now. Get ready, Modest Matildas ... we're going to talk about a few new ways to find those hidden erogenous zones.

If you have trouble with a dry vagina since treatment, try "moisturizing" your vagina daily for a week or two before attempting sexual contact. As Diana Leitch says, "Moisturize your face, moisturize your vagina." Diana gives the example that if you slept all night with your mouth open, the next morning your entire mouth would be incredibly dry, with your tongue feeling thick and probably sticking to the roof of your mouth. You'd have trouble swallowing or placing anything in your mouth. The same holds true for a dry vagina. Placing something into a dry, tight vagina is uncomfortable, painful, and sometimes impossible. Thin vaginal walls can easily tear, which feels like burning and can really hurt! Just as you moisturize your dry skin every night before bed, you can also moisturize a dry vagina every night. (See Chapter Five for more information about using lubricants.) Next, it's time to explore the new you.

"O" MY!
THE ANATOMY OF A FEMALE ORGASM

Woman: An orgasm is a peak of intense pleasure that creates an altered state of consciousness, usually with an explosive initiation, mostly accompanied by involuntary rhythmic vaginal and perineal contractions, sometimes only partially accompanied by a feeling of contentment, which lasts around 12–19 seconds.[1]

Man: It's like scratching an itch that needs scratching.

Many women find it difficult to have an orgasm after cancer treatment, or with menopausal symptoms. What once might have sent waves through your body now provides little pleasure. It's important to understand what happens to your body during an orgasm. It is also essential to note that not all intimate moments must lead to orgasm, and we are not implying an orgasm is the only sexual

> *Many women find it difficult to have an orgasm after cancer treatment, or with menopausal symptoms.*

satisfaction. However, because orgasm can play a role in maintaining a healthy vagina, it's worth an explanation. And besides, it just feels good!

FOUR COUNTS TO LIFT OFF

Masters and Johnson came up with four phases of a woman's sexual response cycle.[2] For our purposes, we have construed these phases to reflect the sexual and intimacy issues that commonly affect women recovering from cancer and its treatment.

Phase One: Excitement. The vagina responds to foreplay by producing moisture or lubrication. Moisture is good, especially when your vagina is dry. The clitoris enlarges with blood and becomes erect. The inside of the vagina might expand, which is good if you have a tight, narrowed vagina. Your heart rate, blood pressure, and muscle tension can all increase during this excitement phase.

Phase Two: Plateau. Between the times you are first aroused until you have an orgasm, the vagina swells and contracts at the vaginal opening. The clitoris shortens, and the inner lips (labia minora) might swell and turn reddish-purple. Again, your blood pressure, muscle tension, and heart rate can rise.

Phase Three: Orgasm. During an orgasm, the pelvic muscles around the vagina and uterus and the anal muscles all contract. Your entire body may spasm, and your blood pressure and heart rate may peak. The contractions that run through your body occur at different times and at different levels of intensity; this provides pleasure during an orgasm.

Phase Four: Resolution. This is the period of time immediately following the orgasm, when your body returns to a normal, relaxed state. During this phase, the blood that engorged your clitoris, inner lips, and vaginal walls flows out, reducing the swelling and muscle tension. This is the time that you'll feel completely relaxed. It's the peaceful "ahhhh" moment when most women want to "cuddle" and most men want to roll over and go to sleep.

During sexual stimulation and orgasm, the vagina is lubricated, blood flows into the area, and the vaginal walls expand, all of which helps maintain the elasticity, tone, and health of the vagina. Sexual stimulation and orgasms are *good for you*. Also during orgasm, a chemical called oxytocin is released. Oxytocin is known as a "bonding" hormone, and it can make you "bond" or feel closer to your lover. It's also important to know that orgasms rarely happen simultaneously; that only happens in the movies.

Did you know orgasms occur in different areas on your body? They don't just happen in your vagina. Some take place in the clitoris, uterus, or entire vulva area. They might feel different, too. For instance, a clitoral orgasm is more focused and intense, whereas a vaginal orgasm is spread more throughout the body. The good news is that if you no longer have orgasms from vaginal stimulation, you can try stimulating another area of your body.

I DID IT ALL BY MYSELF!
VIBRATORS

He said: Why don't you tell me when you have an orgasm?
She said: I would, but you're never there.
(Widespread urban legend and Internet joke)

If your primary erogenous zone was, for instance, your breasts, but they are now numb or missing, you can find new ways to feel sexually satisfied. How do you find those new hot spots? By exploring. For those of you whose religious or cultural beliefs prevent you from self-exploration, we respect your beliefs and also hope that you might consider the benefits of using a vibrator as a medical aid. There are other ways to find new erogenous zones with your partner, which are discussed later in this chapter.

For those of you who would like to explore your body for new sensitive areas, first picture your basic sexual anatomy.

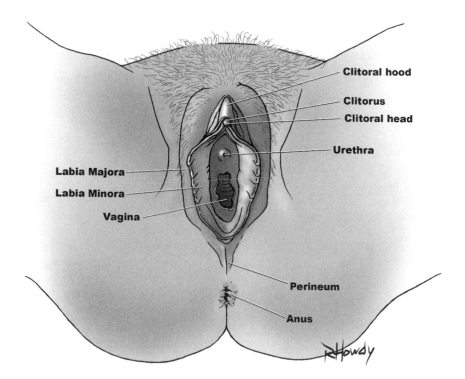

It's important to understand what you are touching so that you can guide your partner to it later, when you are ready. For now, this is your "alone time." You might not be ready for sexual intercourse, emotionally or physically. During this alone time, you can learn what feels good and what doesn't, on your own terms and in your own time.

Remember, using a vibrator for vaginal health is like using a cane to walk when your leg is injured. It is a medical aid. A vibrator helps stretch and maintain the tone of the vagina. You can explore your entire body with the vibrator to determine what feels good now, after cancer treatment. Diana Leitch says, "It's like trying new recipes to find out what you enjoy. The best part is that you can try these new recipes on your own, before sharing them with anyone else, to see what you like."

Exploring new ways to enjoy one another sexually after cancer is wonderful, just remember to keep it gentle and safe. You may want to ask your doctor if using a vibrator or vaginal dilator is right for you before using them. If you are concerned about trying something new, such as a new position, ask your doctor. If you experience vaginal bleeding or pain during sexual contact, be sure to let your doctor know. Your body may not heal the same as it did before cancer, so prevention of injuries and seeking early treatment is critical.

NOTE

Make sure to place plenty of lubrication on the vibrator and in your vagina before attempting to use a vibrator or put anything, including fingers, into the vagina. Make sure the vibrator you choose is one that can be inserted into the vagina; not all vibrators are designed to enter the vagina.

ANNIE, GET YOUR VIBRATOR...

If you have never used a vibrator before, try the following steps to help you get started. Vibrators come in all shapes and sizes. Be gentle while using a vibrator, especially with dry and tissue-thin vaginal walls. What feels good to one person will not work for another, so use your own imagination until you find what works for you. Also, if you do not have a vibrator, you can use your fingers to self-stimulate.

1. **Relax and set the mood.** Take a warm bath, have a glass of wine if you drink, and make sure you have privacy and uninterrupted time set aside. Remove your clothing and get comfortable. You can lie on your bed with your legs bent and slightly apart, or with a pillow under your bent knees. Place the vibrator near you. Make sure to liberally lubricate your vagina and the vibrator first.

2. **Use that big sex organ, your mind.** Think about whatever makes you feel aroused. Recall a past satisfying sexual encounter, a romantic movie, an erotic book, or use your imagination. Turn on your mind... and the vibrator.

3. **Like Columbus on the Mayflower.** Start running your hands and the vibrator lightly over your body to see what feels good. Try different types of touch: a long stroke, a light poke, a pull or pinch, using fingers, the palm of your hand, a vibrator, dildo, or a sex toy. Try to figure out what feels best and where it feels best to be touched. While exploring your body, discover the:

    a. **Clitoris and Inner Lips.** Be sure to only use gentle, mild stimulation (a low-powered vibrator) near your clitoris and your inner lips (labia minora). Also, it is okay to gently place or rub the vibrator against the side of your clitoris and inner lips, but do *not* place the vibrator directly on the head of the clitoris or the inner lips, or you may need to be removed from the ceiling (ouch!). Gently move the vibrator around your clitoris or around your inner lips to see if either are pleasure spots for you.

    b. **Vagina.** You can use a more powerful vibrator directly in the vagina, but remember to lubricate your vagina and the vibrator first. If your vagina is dry and tight, it might help to place only the tip of the vibrator into your vagina and then gently poke it in and out, sort of "teasing" your vagina. (If the vibrator will not go into your vagina, see more information about vaginal dilators in Chapter Five or let your doctor know as there are many causes of vaginal obstruction.)

    c. **Anus.** Some people enjoy anal sex and others do not. Even so, many people enjoy light stimulation of the outside of the anus (or only slightly inside the rectum). While exploring your body, you can use a low-powered vibrator and gently run it over your anus or barely insert the tip into the rectum to see if this is pleasurable for you.

d. **Combo option.** Some women find that a combination of vibrators works best. You can use one hand to insert a vibrator into your vagina. Use the other hand to gently rub a low-powered vibrator on the side of your clitoris at the same time. When and if you decide to engage your partner in using vibrators, he or she can hold a vibrator in one spot and you the other to help you better reach orgasm should this combo work for you.

4. **Hold on when you find it.** When you find an area(s) that feels good, slow down or stop stimulating yourself every now and then to build up excitement. Move your pelvis just like you would during intercourse. Be gentle with yourself. Now is a good time to very carefully thrust the vibrator in and out of your vagina or very gently around your clitoris or inner lips. You can also use your fingers or the palm of your hand, whatever feels best. If your vagina is too narrow, press on the outside of your vagina, or insert only one finger (or see Chapter Five on using a vaginal dilator).

5. **Up, Up, and Away.** If your hands get tired, switch hands or stop moving your hand and let the vibrator do the work. Focus on your breathing if you're having difficulty reaching orgasm. Try breathing fast and hard and then holding your breath for a few seconds. Now is also a good time to do Kegel exercises (see Chapter Five) because the contracting and releasing of those muscles may trigger an orgasm. Continue to caress other parts of your body while you stimulate your vagina or clitoris. You might be surprised to find that having your neck or another area lightly stroked during this time feels erotic. When you begin to feel an orgasm, continue to stimulate yourself in whatever way feels best.

It's possible you won't have an orgasm the first few times you try self-stimulation. The purpose is to find out exactly what feels good and what doesn't. If your vagina is particularly dry, you may not want your partner touching your vagina until you learn through self-stimulation how much lubrication is needed and what positions or touches are pleasant.

Some women worry that they will become "addicted" to a vibrator and prefer it to their partner. To the contrary, many women who stimulate themselves to orgasm find it easier to reach orgasm with their partners and may have sex more frequently. The only reason to prefer a vibrator to a partner is that you've discovered its pleasure. Teach your partner the technique that you discovered.

Exploring on your own can also prevent awkward moments when you're making love with your partner. Because you know what feels good and what doesn't, you can guide your lover to the right areas at the right time and keep your partner from unintentionally hurting you. The way you use a vibrator is a personal preference; each person has unique needs and points of pleasure.

You can purchase a vibrator through a sex therapist, in an adult store or at a sex toy party, or in the privacy of your own home through web sites such as www.mypleasure.com, www.Goodvibes.com, www.babeland.com, or www.xandria.com. No need to worry that your neighbors will see what you're ordering; the vibrators come in plain, unmarked brown envelopes or boxes.

ARE YOU AN "INNY" OR AN "OUTTY"?
(WE'RE NOT TALKING BELLY BUTTONS HERE!)

If you do not want to or are unable to have vaginal intercourse, you and your husband or partner can try "outercourse." This is a term coined by Marty Klein and Riki Robbins in their book, Let Me Count the Ways.[3] It is a great way to bring intimacy back into your relationship without pressure to have intercourse or any kind of sexual contact if you prefer not to. The activities can involve your genitals, or every thing but your genitals. Outercourse assumes that every part of your body is an "erotic zone," and all you have to do is awaken new zones.

Outercourse can assist in rewriting your sexual script, or the rules about who does what and how. You get to be playful and experiment with your mate. You can also go back to very romantic yet nonsexual playfulness. Neither of you should have any expectations about using your "normal" sexual script when experimenting. The only goals are to relax, feel close to one another, and find new ways to feel erotic and sensual.

The first step is to talk with your partner about your desire to reintroduce intimacy or sexuality into your relationship. (See Chapter Eight on ways to communicate about sex.) Talking about sex can be uncomfortable, even for couples who have been together for many years. The point is to break the spiral of not having sex and the silence surrounding this sometimes devastating loss.

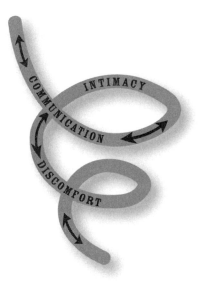

Let your husband or partner know when you are ready to renew a sexual relationship. If you are not ready for intercourse, ask your mate if he is willing to try new ways to become close to you. Outercourse is limited only by your imagination.

The following are a few ways to explore each other sexually or intimately using the concept of outercourse. The first few exercises do not involve genital contact and are wonderful if you want to rebuild intimacy without any pressure for sexual performance.

1. Dance together. Put on your favorite romantic music, dim the lights, eliminate distractions, hold one another, and just dance.

2. Turn off the TV and talk. Sit next to one another and talk about the two of you. No talking about children, bills, or any of the demands of life. Talk about your dreams and hopes together again. You can hold each other during this time if you like.

3. "Make out" with your clothes on as you might have once done as a teenager.

4. Cuddle together and hold each other for a long time. You can do this while wearing your clothes or while naked.

5. Give each other a massage. Use scented oils or lotions if you like, as long as they are safe and appropriate for you.

6. Shower together. Slowly lather up your mate and run your hands over each other's bodies.

7. Have phone sex or Internet sex. Talk about what you would like to do to each other sexually.

8. Use your fingers to feed each other your favorite foods. This can bring laughter and surprisingly erotic feelings if you do this while closely staring at one another.

For those of you who are ready for more sexual or genital contact that does not include intercourse, try the following outercourse activities.

1. Rub lotion or oil on just one of you. Then have that naked person slide or rub all over the other naked person with his or her body.

2. Kiss every place on your partner's body *except* the lips.

3. Use a vibrator on one another. If you haven't used a vibrator before, it's a good idea to first practice using one alone. Many heterosexual

men feel more comfortable using a vibrator that does not look like a penis, so you might keep that in mind when ordering vibrators if you want to use them with your partner.

4. Have oral sex. If your vagina is too dry for intercourse, oral sex can be very pleasing, especially if your partner focuses on your clitoris and not necessarily your vagina. Your partner also benefits from this type of sexual contact without the need for intercourse.

5. Masturbate one another. Again, make sure to first lubricate your vagina and your partner's fingers when masturbating. Make sure your partner is careful when touching your genitals. You may also ask your partner to masturbate other areas of your body that do not involve your genitals.

6. Masturbate yourselves while looking into each other's eyes. This can promote deep intimacy and closeness in your sexual relationship. You can also avoid any discomfort from your partner unintentionally touching a painful spot on your body.

These are just a few suggestions for outercourse. Only your imagination limits you and your lover. Outercourse is a wonderful option when you are either unable to or no longer desire intercourse. Sex does not have to involve your genitals. Finding new sensual ways to feel close with your partner allows you to feel accepted, comfortable with your body, confident, and close to your partner. Many people experience orgasms during outercourse. You can still have an active sexual life without intercourse.

UP, UP, AND AWAY!
...AND OTHER SEXUAL POSITIONS

In life, being on top is generally easier...this goes for sexual intercourse too! When you are positioned on top of your husband or partner, you have more control over the amount of sexual penetration. It's also possible a penis can glide more easily into the vagina when you're on top. This is really important if you have a dry, tight vagina or thin, narrow vaginal walls after cancer treatment. If your vagina completely loses elasticity, the stretching needed to accommodate sexual intercourse will not return. Again, use it or lose it. This is why maintaining an active sex life, whether with your partner or through self-stimulation, is so important. Keeping your vagina lubricated with moisture and stimulated with blood flow can keep it healthy and toned.

> *If intercourse is painful, or if you have been unable to succeed with intercourse after cancer treatment, a different sexual position might help.* ❖

If intercourse is painful, or if you have been unable to succeed with intercourse after cancer treatment, a different sexual position might help. An alternative position may also help you discover new ways to feel pleasure. Experiment, but be gentle. This is not the time to have wild, passionate sex. Gentle, careful penetration will prevent tears, pain, and discomfort during intercourse.

In addition to the missionary position, a few other positions that may alleviate pain or allow you to succeed with intercourse are shown on the next two pages.

Try one position, and if it doesn't work, try another. Again, be gentle and remember to use plenty of lubrication on both you and your partner before attempting intercourse.

Another option is a technique called coital alignment (see the sexual position that uses a pillow under her bottom). A man positions himself to "ride a little higher" than normal so that his penis is at more of a 90-degree angle, which stimulates the clitoris as it enters the vagina. This is supposed to increase the likelihood of female orgasm. While your husband or partner positions himself a little higher up toward your belly, you should elevate your hips (you can use a pillow to prop your hips higher), which makes the experience more comfortable and allows the two of you to work together toward orgasm.

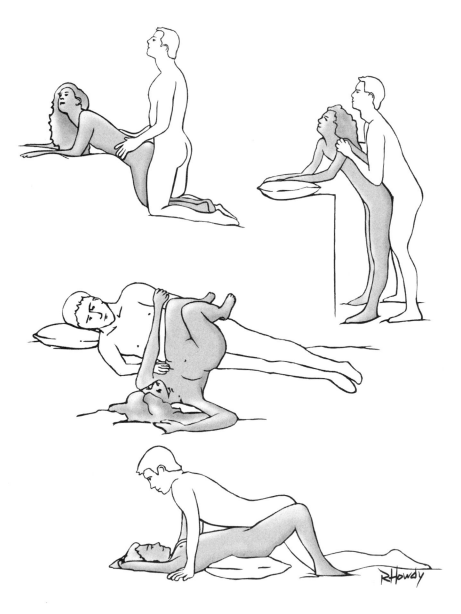

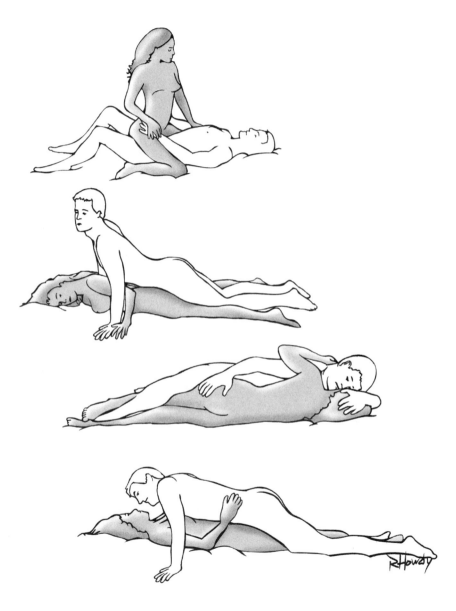

A ROAD LESS TRAVELED?
SENSATE FOCUS

My wife and I have the secret to making a marriage last. Two times a week, we go to a nice restaurant, have a little wine, good food. She goes on Tuesdays, and I go on Fridays.
(Widely spread urban legend and Internet joke)

When you are ready, you can come together to build a stronger intimate and sexual life with your lover by exploring new erogenous zones together. Sensate focus is one way to explore sexual touch. Masters & Johnson came up with the technique called "sensate focus" in the 1960s.[4] The idea is that neither of you expect to have intercourse or even become sexually aroused when you begin. This takes off any pressure to perform sexually. Sensate focus allows you to relax and focus on the pure pleasure of sexual touch. The exercises can be quite helpful when you are ready to reawaken sexuality but have avoided intimacy for fear it would lead to intercourse.

There are three basic steps involved in sensate focus. It is extremely important that you set aside enough uninterrupted time to complete these exercises. Otherwise, you'll feel anxious and unable to enjoy the time together. For your first session, set aside at least one hour of private time with your lover.

STEP ONE: BODY CARESSES

Each of you takes a turn being the giver and the receiver. When you are the receiver, your spouse or partner begins by touching your naked body every place *except* your breasts (or the place where your breasts used to be) and your genitals. If you are self-conscious about your body because of breast reconstruction or missing breasts, you may want to begin this exercise by wearing a sexy bra or lingerie. Eventually, you can remove your top when you become more comfortable with your partner seeing this area.

To start, lie on your stomach. You can use scented oils or lotions during this step. For at least 15 minutes, your partner should touch the back of your body by lightly stroking all areas of your backside. During this time, try to remove all thoughts from your mind and concentrate on the touching and the sensations you are feeling. Think about what feels good as your lover strokes your backside.

After 15 minutes, turn over on your back. For the next 15 minutes, your partner should stroke and touch the front of your body, *except* for your breasts and genitals. Again, remove all thoughts from your mind except the sensation of being touched. Think about what feels good and what doesn't. You should not speak during this time, unless it is to tell your partner when something does *not* feel good. Try not to moan or make sounds when your partner does stroke areas that feel good, because your partner should continue to explore your entire body and not focus on one stimulated area.

After 30 minutes of touch, change places with your partner. You become the "giver" and your husband or partner becomes the "receiver." Repeat the same process as above. During this stage, you and your lover tune in to your bodies with sensual touch. You may feel sexually and intimately connected to one another when you complete this step. At the end of the exercise, both of you should tell each other what parts of the experience were the most pleasurable. You can continue to the next step the following day or repeat step one a few more times on other days before moving on.

STEP TWO – SENSUAL TOUCH WITHOUT ORGASM

During this second exercise, your partner again gently touches or strokes your entire body, only this time, your lover can stroke your breasts, or the place where your breasts used to be, and your genitals. The focus should not just be on your breasts and genitals, however. You also should not focus on his genitals either. Again, one of you is the giver and one is the receiver for 30 minutes each. During that time, each of you should focus on the entire body of your lover. You each can briefly stroke or lightly touch genitals and breasts, but do not remain touching these areas for more than a minute or two at a time. Do not bring one another to orgasm during this exercise. If you or your partner begins to become very aroused, stop touching the area that is causing the arousal and move to another area of the body. It is okay to briefly return to these sensitive areas, but do not remain there or trigger an orgasm.

During this step, you and your partner can give each other more guidance during the sensual touching about what feels good. You can either quietly verbalize "put your hand there," or "touch me this way," or you can gently guide your partner's hand to the area and show him how to touch you in a way that is pleasurable; he can do the same when you are the giver and he is the receiver.

This exercise helps you discover how to enjoy genital caressing without the pressure of performing or having an orgasm. This step is more sexually stimulating or exciting than step one, but neither of you should expect to have intercourse or an orgasm. You're simply enjoying one another's bodies in a relaxed way without anxiety or demands.

Step Three – Sensual Touch, Orgasm Optional

During this step, more focus is paid to the genitals and breasts (if your breasts are numb, find other erotic or sensual areas through exploration). Again, each of you takes turns being the giver and receiver. Start by lying on your stomach and receiving sensual touch on your backside. Then turn over to receive sensual touch on the front of your body. Each of you can spend most of the time on the genitals and other newly discovered sensual areas of one another's bodies if you like.

During this exercise, either of you may choose to continue to be caressed until you have an orgasm. If you are not ready to have an orgasm, ask your partner to stop touching the areas that are highly stimulating for you and move to other parts of your body. Your partner can return to that area for a brief time to arouse you and then, once again, stop short of causing an orgasm. The purpose of this step is to feel pleasure with sexual touch, not necessarily orgasm.

If you are both open to oral sex, now is a good time to include it if you wish. Also, many couples do end up enjoying intercourse at the end of this exercise. Again, this is entirely up to you. The purpose of sensate focus is to awaken your senses to other types of sexual pleasure, but it is perfectly acceptable to end the exercises with intercourse when you are ready.

Keeping an Open Mind

There are many ways to feel sexual pleasure. After cancer treatment, you may need to explore different ways to enjoy sex, perhaps in ways that you had not thought of before. While you may be sexually frustrated or even worried about rekindling your sexual life, experimenting with someone you love can be wonderful and exciting. Keep an open mind. Ask your partner to keep an open mind. The more sexual activity you participate in, the more likely you will preserve your sexual functioning. When you are ready and after you've had a chance to determine what feels good now, the two of you can rewrite your sexual script together.

Be sure to remove outside stressors, schedule quiet time together, communicate about what feels good and what doesn't, and let your partner know if you would rather not be touched just yet. Don't be afraid to experiment. Vaginal intercourse is not the only way to achieve sexual pleasure. It's a new day. It's a new you. It's a new journey!

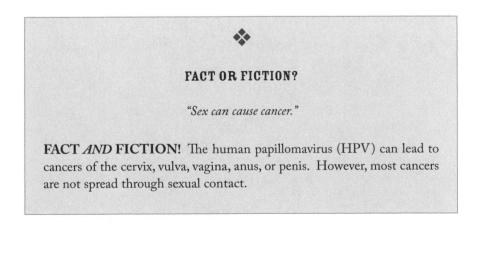

❖

FACT OR FICTION?

"Sex can cause cancer."

FACT *AND* FICTION! The human papillomavirus (HPV) can lead to cancers of the cervix, vulva, vagina, anus, or penis. However, most cancers are not spread through sexual contact.

[1] Basson R, Leiblum S, et al. (2004). Revised Definitions of Womens' Sexual Dysfunctions. <u>The Journal of Sexual Medicine</u>, 1(1), pp. 40-48.

[2] Masters WH, Johnson VE (1966). <u>Human Sexual Response</u>. Boston: Little, Brown. (Lippincott Williams & Wilkins Publishers. ISBN 0316549878.)

[3] Klein M, Robbins R (1998). <u>What is Outercourse? Let Me Count the Ways</u>, Ch. 3, pp. 114-116. New York: Jeremy P. Tarcher/Putnam.

[4] Masters & Johnson, <u>supra</u>, n. 1.

EIGHT

He Said, She Said

NOTE

While same-sex partners also have sexual communication issues, there are indications you may be more open to voicing your concerns. For that reason, this chapter focuses on communication between men and women but does not exclude same-sex relationships.

> *My wife says I never listen to her...*
> *At least I think that's what she said.*
>
> *(Widely spread Internet joke)*

ommunication between the sexes has been troublesome since the first man and woman became a couple.

> ***Eve:*** *What are you thinking about, Adam?*
> ***Adam:*** *(Staring intensely at nothing) Huh? Oh, I was just wondering if I could take the fur from an animal to clothe us. These fig leaves are itchy.*

> **Eve:** *Oh, you think I look fat in this fig leaf, don't you?*
> **Adam:** *Whuh?*
> **Eve:** *I knew it! You want to cover me up with fur because you're not attracted to me anymore!*

After cancer treatment, an altered body and the side effects of treatment can introduce new or additional sexual problems into your relationship. Most of us don't feel comfortable discussing sex. In fact, it may be easier for some to talk about dying than it is to talk about sex with your partner. Sex is taboo, a mystical thing we tend to figure out on our own. We're not *supposed* to talk about sex. Most couples don't regularly discuss the quality of their sex lives, regardless of having had cancer. If you were one of the unique couples who freely talked about sex before cancer, your road to returning to an active sex life may be a little smoother. However, most of us fall into the *other* category, where communicating about sexual problems is a winding road with many potholes.

Begin this journey by asking yourself a few questions. Is your voice being heard? Are you listening to your partner's concerns? What assumptions are you making about your partner's thoughts or behaviors since your diagnosis? Are these notions accurate, or might you be projecting your fears and self-esteem issues onto his quiet or unusual behavior? The fact of the matter is that your partner, if he is at all supportive or loving, has been fighting your cancer too – *with* you. It's true that the cancer happened to *you,* *your* body, and *your* life. Yet it's possible your husband or partner might have been more frightened or worried about this battle than you have imagined.

A SPOUSE OR A LOUSE...
GOT BUG SPRAY?

It's normal to struggle with accepting an altered or disfigured body along with the other side effects of cancer and its treatment. Your husband or partner's response to these changes may not have been what you had hoped. While there are varying degrees of acceptable behavior in your mate, there is a difference between being a quiet, supportive husband and a louse.

> *I was 32 when I was diagnosed with uterine cancer. My husband was too busy to attend doctor appointments or care for me after surgery and chemotherapy. I stayed with my mother. While he asked about my progress, he seemed annoyed when I told him details. After I recovered, I left him. While it was painful at the time, I later realized he had never been a giving partner. It's been six years, and I've never felt happier.*
>
> Stacy*, 38

If you are with someone who makes you feel worse (and not better) about yourself since cancer treatment, it's time to bring in other support. Friends, family, adult children, cancer support groups, and spiritual or other professional counselors are all options for providing the support you need and deserve. Some women discover they no longer want to put up with a partner who is critical, unkind, or worse. Keep in mind, however, that it's possible you might be misinterpreting his fearful behavior as a lack of concern. Talking with an objective person(s) may help you decide into which category your relationship falls.

SUPERMAN AND WONDER WOMAN
BOTH SUPERHEROES, DIFFERENT COMIC BOOKS

In an intimate relationship, we might assume that the two of us are concerned about similar issues and priorities; however, it's possible that we have very different views of what is important. It's possible he is focused on one aspect of the marriage or partnership and you another. You may be focused on the intimate aspects of the relationship while he

Most men are not as concerned as women are about women's altered bodies after cancer.

is focused on making sure you don't have to worry about finances. While worrying about intimacy, you might be concerned about his reaction to your missing breast(s) or the addition of an ostomy bag since men are basically visual beings. *Attention: Most men are not as concerned as women are about women's altered bodies after cancer.* Regardless of what you think he is thinking, his primary concern is likely that you are alive and well. The change to your body or loss of any body part, including the breast, is usually meaningless to him (unless, of course, he is a louse).

> *I want her well and here with me. I don't care about her missing breasts. She's more than two breasts or two arms or two legs. I just want the cancer gone.*
>
> William*, 44

> *I know she is grieving the loss of her breasts, and that the reconstructed breasts are not the same. When she asks me what I think of them, I don't know what to say. They are beautiful. She is beautiful. I am so glad she is here with me. But I know she misses her real breasts; we both do. If I say it doesn't matter, then she tells me of course it does and says I'm insensitive. If I tell her I miss her breasts too, she feels less than the woman I married. I don't know what to say.*
>
> Dan*, 55

> *It's true…the first thing I noticed about my girlfriend were her breasts. Breasts really turn me on, and I feel so terrible that I miss them. But I would miss her more. I really love this woman. She is supposed to have reconstructive surgery soon. She teases me she is going to get bigger breasts than she had before. We both know her new breasts will be numb, but she says she'll let me touch them anyway! If it turns out she can't have reconstructive surgery, I've heard we can we find other erogenous zones. I'm all for it.*
>
> Anthony*, 36

Even if your partner can't express it, he may be thinking similar thoughts as these men. Yet if neither of you is talking about sexual issues, how can you really know what the other is thinking? The trick is to start talking. But how?

Women are better than men with the "I feel" discussions. Men have to first really get in touch with this part of their brains. Women and men basically see the world differently. Men are usually more in tune with the spatial part of a relationship or how things work together as a whole. Women are more inclined to see the details of a relationship, or how one part of a relationship fits together with or influences another part.

Men are generally more concerned about seeing results or "fixing" a problem. They don't want a lot of "jibber jabber," but want to get to the bottom line quickly, and identify the problem that needs to be "fixed." Women, on the other hand, want to work through the problem by talking about it. We love communication, sharing, and agreement in our relationships. These differences make you wonder how we ever come together on important relationship matters! But we can and we do.

If you have trouble communicating with your partner, you're not alone. How can you really know what he is thinking about your relationship since cancer? How do you make sure he understands exactly what you now want and need?

Be specific. Don't make him guess what you are feeling or thinking, and then punish him because he is too "dense" to know this on his own. When a man says he doesn't know what you want, chances are he truly doesn't know what you want. It doesn't necessarily mean he isn't interested in finding out.

A man won't understand what your sexual needs are unless you tell him exactly what those needs are in a way he will understand. If you can verbalize your sexual needs to your partner, and he can communicate the same to you, the two of you can have a healthy sexual relationship. It sounds simple, but it isn't always so easy. Make sure your partner understands that you will not judge him for expressing his needs or how he is feeling about the relationship. Reassure him that there is no right or wrong answer as you both question what it is each of you wants now. Remember, men like to identify and solve problems. It's how you relay your concerns to him that is important. Sometimes, the solutions simply won't come easily, which can frustrate both of you.

Sex is not a cure. For some reason, men often think sex will make everything better. From a woman's perspective, sex takes time and energy. A woman has to be present emotionally during sex. A man is relaxed by sex. If he's had a stressful day, having sex may reduce the stress. After a stressful day, a woman often prefers sleep to sex.

One man whose wife was recovering from breast cancer continued to goad her for sex, saying, "Come on, honey, it will make you feel better." Make sure your partner understands that "No" means no. If you don't want to have sex yet, it's essential for you to communicate that clearly to your husband or partner. Make sure you let him know what is going on inside your heart, mind, and body so he understands your lack of desire is not about him, but about where you are emotionally and physically. Emotion plays a role in a woman's need for sex. Again, be clear about what you want and don't want. For example, say "I just need you to hold me without it going any further," if that is what you want. When a woman asks, "Honey, come here and hold me," a man may hear, "Honey, come here and [screw] me." Men don't always understand the difference. You may have to explain to him in detail exactly what you are ready for and what you are not ready for in your love life.

On the other hand, many men, when shown exactly what needs to happen, respond beautifully. For instance, one woman's husband took outstanding care of her but only *after* a nurse showed him exactly what to do – down to explicit instructions such as "put your forearms under her arms to lift her…place her on this part of the bed…lift her legs," and so on. Sometimes men may need step-by-step instructions about intimacy and sex.

A lot of things have changed since your diagnosis. You are probably not the same person you were when you heard the words, "You have cancer." He has likely changed too. You also can't assume you know what he is thinking or feeling, especially if he has withdrawn or become more quiet since your diagnosis and treatment. He may be trying to figure out how he can "fix" the situation, unsure of what either of you wants or needs. Open communication can lead toward working together to identify each other's needs. The most important relationship in your lives can be stronger and better than ever.

I'LL LOVE YOU FOREVER...
WHO ARE YOU ANYWAY?

Mike and his wife June attended a marriage seminar dealing with communication. The instructor explained, "It is vital that husbands and wives know the things that are important to each other." He addressed Mike, "What is your wife's favorite flower?"

Mike leaned over and whispered to his wife, "It's Pillsbury, isn't it, honey?"

(Widely spread urban legend and Internet joke)

Sometimes we get into a comfortable pattern in our long-term love affair. Yet even without the invasion of cancer, we each grow as individuals over the years, develop new interests, passions, and inspirations. For instance, you both might have started out listening to rock music together but now you like opera, and he likes country. Sometimes we grow together as a couple, and sometimes that growth takes place at different times and in different directions. How did the two of you grow together or apart during your cancer diagnosis and treatment? Women who were treated for cancer share the following common thoughts about their central relationship. Here are some of the typical quotes we heard in the course of researching this book:

We have a happy marriage, but haven't had sex in years. I would like to, but my husband lost interest when I was diagnosed. After being turned down, I don't ask him anymore.

Chemo left me uninterested in sex, and we don't attempt sex often.

My partner left after my chemo was over, so I suppose he was turned off by my appearance. I feel so unattractive. Who will want me now?

My husband is in love with all of me, warts and all.

When cancer and its treatment interfere with intimacy and sex, how do the two of you talk about it? Learning to discuss sex with your lover is a crucial step toward reclaiming a satisfying sex life after cancer treatment. Unfortunately, talking openly about sex, even in long-term marriages or loving relationships, is difficult for most of us, especially if we didn't talk openly about it before.

As you know, our culture, body image and self-esteem all play enormous roles in how we view and talk about sex and intimacy. What words come to mind when you hear the word "sex"? What words come to mind when you hear the words "great sex"? Many of the women in Dr. Kydd's workshops described great sex as "vacation sex." Most of us would tend to agree. But what makes it great? How about no distractions (such as freedom from childcare responsibilities), little if any stress, lots of foreplay, and plenty of time for each other, relaxation, and meaningful communication. Vacation sex is about romance, cuddling afterwards, and taking the time to truly make love. We can have that kind of lovemaking at home, too.

COMMUNICATION STYLES

Every couple has a preferred communication style or comfort zone when talking about sex. Knowing your communication style could help ignite the conversation. Dr. Leslie Schover, in her book, <u>Sexuality and Fertility After Cancer,</u> describes four basic communication styles when it comes to talking about sex.[1] For our purpose, we interpret these characteristics with our own titles and ask: Are you a "silent type", a "predictable partner", a "sexual gourmet", or a "fighter, not a lover"?

Silent Types. If you are uncomfortable talking about sex, you're probably the silent type. Perhaps neither of you has much experience with sex, and you don't talk about sex, especially with each other. You learn about each other's bodies through trial and error and do not ask for what you want. Sex may not be satisfying. After cancer treatment, you might quickly give up on sex if you can't fall back into old routines.

Predictable Partners. The two of you talk only occasionally about sex, and your communication style and your sexual interactions may be predictable. You don't discuss sex often, and you probably have fallen into a relaxed routine of lovemaking that lacks variety. One person usually initiates sex more often. Sex is not the most important aspect of your relationship. When cancer enters the picture, you may lack the skills to communicate openly.

A Sexual Gourmet. If you fit into this category, sex was a central part of your relationship. Just as food gourmets enjoy talking about food, and enjoy experiencing a variety of foods, a sexual gourmet enjoys discussing sex and sexual variety. You might freely discuss what each of you enjoys and spend a great deal of time making love or "feasting" on your sexual pleasures. However, once one of you loses desire or the "ability to enjoy the feast," you both become lost. Your partner may feel inadequate, annoyed, hurt, or confused that you no longer share an interest in sex.

A Fighter, Not a Lover. If you argue about sex, you probably fit into this category. Here, sex has always been a troubled subject. Often, you blame each other for problems in your sex life or for the lack of lovemaking. Also, each of you may retain anger, grudges, or hostility toward the other person that has nothing to do with sex, but you bring these resentments into the bedroom. Losing your libido only increases the frustration and anger surrounding your partner and your sex life.

Once you are able to identify your communication style, the two of you can work toward a more open, healthy way of talking about sexual challenges since cancer treatment. Like the old saying goes: You can't know where you're going if you don't know where you're coming from.

HAPPY TALKING HAPPY TALK?

A husband read an article to his wife about how many words women use each day – 30,000 to a man's 15,000. The wife said, "That's because we have to repeat everything we say to men." The husband turned to his wife and said, "What?"
(Widely spread urban legend and Internet joke)

How do you move toward open communication, especially about sex, when men and women think and respond so differently? When bringing up the conversation about sex, you might try using the "Talking rules."

Rule 1: Talk outside the bedroom. Schedule a private time to talk when neither of you is exhausted or feeling stressed. Do not attempt to have this talk during sex or foreplay. If you have children, ask someone else to take care of them so you won't be interrupted. Take the phone off the hook if needed.

Rule 2: Talk about the weather. Get comfortable with general conversation first. It's best not to jump right into tough talk about big problems. Spend a few minutes quietly and kindly talking with one another. Set the tone in the beginning for the rest of the conversation.

Rule 3: Talk about one or two issues. Instead of exploring every hurt, concern, or problem in your love life, try focusing on just one or two. You can discuss other concerns another time. Remember to also discuss solutions. For example, you might tell him that you need more intimate, loving touches that do not lead to sex. He might tell you he feels closest to you when you make love. The solution could be that he agrees to express more non-sexual attention toward you during the week, while you commit to making love every Saturday night. The result is that each of you gets what you want and need: you feel more relaxed and enjoy his touches during the week, and he looks forward to the weekend.

Rule 4: Talk about what works. Try not to criticize the other person. Tell what the other is doing *right* as well as identifying what needs improvement. When he does something right when you are intimate, praise him for it. Talk about what feels good and what doesn't. A lack of non-sexual intimacy also has consequences to your sex life. Women need to feel close or emotionally connected to their lover in order to enjoy sex.

> *Women need a reason and men need a place for sex. Women need a place and men need a reason for communication.*
>
> *Dr. Sally Kydd*

Rule 5: Talk about "I," not "You." You can avoid arguments by telling your mate how you feel about something specific instead of criticizing him. For instance, say, "I feel rejected because you don't try to make love to me anymore" rather than, "You aren't attracted to me." Agree to be gentle with one another in conversation. Don't blame one another, and make a point of staying on the topic you're discussing without bringing other issues into the conversation. Make positive suggestions about changing your sex life.

Rule 6: Talk, and then listen – even if he's quiet. The biggest misconception we have as women when communicating with men is that we believe they are not listening to us when they remain quiet. We feel ignored when a man doesn't respond to our words. Rest assured, he hears you. However, while continuing to talk without letting him respond may allow us to release pent-up emotions, it may also cause him to build a protective wall while he processes what you've said. This is why it is vital to take turns talking and to limit each scheduled talk to one or two items at a time, even if your list is a mile long. Walking that mile begins with the first step: communication.

Women need to express themselves, while men feel nagged by too many words. According Dr. Deborah Tannen in <u>You Just Don't Understand: Women and Men in Conversation,</u> only women try to establish a connection by communicating. Men seek to establish dominance or a chain of command (hierarchy).[2]

In "My Fair Lady," Henry Higgins poses the question, "Why can't a woman be more like a man?" Yet many women would like just the opposite in their intimate relationship; women would love to see men become more like them when it comes to communication.

Rule 7: Talk about his concerns. It's imperative to get feedback from your husband or partner during this discussion. Make eye contact with him, don't cross your arms, and do not interrupt. You might want to limit the time to two to three minutes each when one of you speaks and the other does not interrupt. Ask him what he thinks about your sex life. When it is your turn to talk, rephrase what he said before you give feedback so he knows he's been heard and so you are sure you understand what he said. He should do the same for you. Keep in mind that he might have been resisting making love to you because he thought you already had enough to deal with. One man told us it was difficult to make love to someone who had been so very ill. You may have to encourage him to express his concerns. Be prepared to wait for him to gather his thoughts. Remember, men generally talk in conclusions, not itemized lists.

Rule 8: Talk about your fears. Tell him your concerns about sex and your relationship, using the words, "I feel" this or that and not, "You do this," or, "You don't ever do that." You may have fears about being rejected sexually by him, especially if your body has been altered by treatment. You may also fear that your marriage is in trouble if you have lost intimacy (not just sex) in your relationship. You may have other fears related to your cancer treatment, such as whether you are now capable of making love or whether you are now infertile. The return of cancer may be your greatest fear. All of these concerns are legitimate, whether or not they prove true, and all of your concerns deserve attention. Unresolved emotions interrupt the healthy flow of a sexual and intimate relationship.

Now that you know the ground rules, you can schedule the conversation when you are ready. It might first help to know a little bit more about common mistakes we make when communicating.

MISTAKING HIS SILENCE FOR AGREEMENT

Cancer doesn't happen when it's convenient. It's *never* convenient for cancer to invade your life. There are jobs to keep, bills to pay, meals to prepare, and all of the other normal challenges that life throws your way. Then comes cancer, poking its ugly head into your affairs and turning life upside down.

When I was diagnosed with breast cancer, my husband had just accepted a new important position with a large company. He was bombarded by all the stressful changes associated with a new job. While he was concerned about me, he seemed to be much more focused on his new career than he was on my doctor appointments. He wasn't exactly there for me, holding my hand at every turn. I resented the hell out of him for that. My resentment crept into our bedroom, and our sex life was awful for a really long time after my recovery. It wasn't until I was able to express to him that I had felt abandoned that things resolved. He told me he had felt completely powerless to help me, so he focused on what he could control, and that was making sure I was provided for.

Sydney*, 51

HIS SILENCE = HE AGREES I'M DAMAGED GOODS

Her Diary: He was quiet and seemed distant when he picked me up. I thought he was angry with me because I took so long to get ready. We didn't speak much during dinner, and I asked if we could find a quiet place to talk. He remained sullen and quiet. When I asked, "What's wrong?" he would only say, "Nothing." I asked if he was angry with me for being late. He said, "No." I said, "I love you," but he just smiled at me but said nothing.

He remained silent and distant, and I finally went to bed by myself. He followed me in a little while later and wanted to make love, yet he was still distant and seemed to be thinking about something else the whole time. I couldn't stand it anymore, started crying, and leaned over to ask him again what was wrong. By this time, he had fallen fast asleep. I cried all night long because I knew he didn't really love me anymore. I was convinced he was having an affair. I'm not sure what I'll do. My life is over.

His Diary: Today my favorite football team lost the big game, but at least I got laid.

(Widely spread urban legend and Internet joke)

Don't interpret his silence as rejection. A woman assumes her husband or partner is rejecting her when he doesn't attempt to touch her sexually. This is frequently not the case after cancer. You might feel insecure about your changed appearance since treatment. He might still be in the caretaker or protector mode of seeing you as a person who has been very ill. You might need his touches, kisses, and sweet talk. He might worry you will interpret his tenderness as pushing you into having sex when you're not ready. More than anything, he may be worried he will hurt you physically if he attempts to make love to you. He may be waiting for you to tell him clearly and specifically that you want to try making love again. If you aren't ready for intercourse but want sexual contact, you'll have to be specific with him about what you want. Ask him what he wants too. And remind him that until you're ready, "No" means no.

Men generally don't ask for directions when they are lost. Instead, men focus on what needs to be done to get back on course. They might wander for quite some time before seeing a road they recognize, or before they turn onto the path that takes them back to the right road. Why do you think it took Moses 40 years to get out of the desert? During this time of wandering, men will be unlikely to admit they don't know where they are or where they are going. Men are just determined to get there, and in the fastest time possible. You may be the one to provide the directions to get your love life back on course. This can only happen if you talk about it.

A husband and wife had an argument and were giving each other the silent treatment. Just before bedtime, the man suddenly realized he needed his wife to wake him for an early business meeting. Not wanting to be the first to break the silence, he wrote a note to his wife, "Please wake me at 5:00 a.m." and left the note where she would find it.

The next morning, the man woke up at 8:00 a.m. and realized he'd missed his business meeting. He was furious with his wife and was about to go find her when he saw her note by his side of the bed. Her note read, "It's 5:00 a.m. Wake up."
(Widely spread urban legend and Internet joke)

BEGIN THE BEGINNING

Where to begin…especially when you're not comfortable talking about sex. "Meta-communication" is a term used to describe when you "talk" about "talking about" a subject (before you actually discuss the actual subject). If discussing your sex life is too difficult, then begin by simply talking together about the *idea of talking* about your sex life. This initial discussion may not be so frightening for either of you. Then, if you can get through this chat, or if neither of you has a problem discussing your sex life, you can schedule the date to talk about it.

If discussing your sex life is too difficult, then begin by simply talking together about the idea of talking about your sex life.

Ask your husband or partner to meet you at a specific time and place for an hour or two. If you are comfortable with it, tell him you want to talk with him about where your sex life is headed. If either of you is uncomfortable with this topic, then just tell him you would like to meet to talk about the changes you've both been through since your diagnosis and treatment.

If either of you is extremely uncomfortable discussing sex or intimacy issues, try writing down your issues in a letter. Again, use the same "talking" guidelines outlined above. No accusations, only discuss a few items at a time, and tell him you want to hear from him about his concerns too. Have a special place or "love mailbox" where you place the letters to each other. Read them when you are each ready, together or separately. It's possible you may begin your conversations in writing and then eventually be able to talk about them face-to-face. Give it time. If you've been the silent types, it may take a little while to find your new comfort zone.

Some couples find they are more uninhibited about dealing with sexual issues while making love. It's okay for you to place his hand where you want it during lovemaking, but you probably don't want to delve into a discussion of sexual issues at this time. Talking about your sex life when you are making love can be a "passion-killer." This is an especially bad time to discuss sexual frustrations for the couple who fits into the "I'm A Fighter, Not A Lover" communication style.

LOOK WHAT WE DONE, MA!
EXPECT SOME POSITIVE RESULTS
FROM OPEN COMMUNICATION

After my mastectomy, I was very concerned about my husband seeing my scar. I was quite a sight…one breast red and tight from radiation and one breast missing. When I actually got up the courage to tell my husband about my concerns, he said to me, "Oh honey, you're every man's dream – it's like being with two women at one time!"

Becky Olson

Just think, with a little communication, you may be able to set aside your fears or concerns about your lover's reaction to your new body. It's important to remember that many different emotions surface after cancer, including a passion for life and the fear of dying or of recurrence; it's tough to sort them all out. It's sometimes difficult to know where the feelings are coming from. These feelings happen to your partner, too. He may be afraid of hurting you or simply unsure how to react to the changes in you. Neither of you may know what the changes are or how to deal with them. Talking about them can break down any barriers that may have developed between you.

You have likely gone from thinking, "Will I die," or, "I'm going to beat this illness" when you were ill to more typical daily thoughts, including thoughts about your love life as you begin to feel better. Returning to a routine or "normal" life is a long journey. Struggling to keep your fears under control can suppress other emotions, too. Many women stop feeling much of anything, and mention how numb they feel sexually as well.

Cancer doesn't select only the few who can handle it; cancer happens to both weak and strong relationships. When it occurs in an already weakened relationship, it simply has to get in line behind many other problems. Cancer can break up marriages that are already too weak to handle another crisis. In some instances, cancer is the catalyst that makes a woman look honestly at her life to decide if this relationship is really what she wants. Some women decide this is not the life they want and now is the time to make a change.

On the other hand, there are also many good, loving men out there who want to help but don't know how. Men are often uncomfortable with strong emotions. It is not necessarily "natural" for them to deal with these emotions. They have often been raised to be strong, to provide for their family, and to leave emotional concerns to the women in their lives. They usually try to fix a problem so they don't have to feel strong emotions.

Kathy LaTour, cancer survivor and author of a wonderful book, <u>The Breast Cancer Companion</u>, says, "Men know how to either fix it, kill it, or sue it." Yet Kathy points out that some women also have difficulty communicating their strong emotions after cancer.

> *I have moved into the shadow of the valley of death and hung curtains and now live here. It's difficult for the other person to come and live with you there.*
>
> *Kathy LaTour*

When Kathy was diagnosed with cancer, sex was never discussed by her doctors or with her partner. The focus was on living. "After four years into recovery, I began to understand that I had done the medical side of cancer really well, but I had not done the heart part well." Kathy had not looked at the way cancer was affecting who she was as a person. "Now that I had embraced cancer and the fear of dying, it affected every aspect of my life." Kathy found help in a support group to work through the emotional issues wrought by cancer. She suggests women go someplace where they can talk about their feelings, because for women, those feelings and sexual desire are connected.

A woman who had a double mastectomy and reconstructive surgery provides another example of something really special that resulted from good communication. When her husband no longer touched her breasts during foreplay, she felt rejected and hurt; yet she wouldn't have felt a thing if he had touched her breasts because they were completely numb. Still, her resentment rose from what she perceived as his rejection. Finally, she got up the courage to ask her husband why he didn't pay attention to her breasts anymore. His response set her free:

I only ever paid attention to your breasts because I knew they gave you pleasure during lovemaking. I didn't do it for me, darling, I did it for you. Now that they don't give you pleasure, there's no reason for me to touch them.

John*, 60

It's also important to note that even when a woman is in the end stages of cancer, intimacy is crucial to her. The Canadian Breast Cancer Network (CBCN) surveyed women in the last stages of cancer and found that touching, caressing, kissing, and sometimes sexual intercourse were still very important. We are all beings who need intimacy to feel connected and alive.

Loss of interest in sex and intimacy is like the proverbial elephant in the room. Everyone knows it's there, but the beast is hardly ever acknowledged. The great physical and psychological losses surrounding your intimate life are often not discussed; or maybe worse, they are consciously ignored. Some of us don't even discuss our concerns with our partners or our doctors. It's imperative that you find your voice in all of this. The loss of your sex drive or your ability to perform is neither a "dirty little secret," nor does it mean there is something wrong with you. On the contrary, this lack of discussion is a missing cog in our culture and in our health care system.

Now that you have a few tools to begin talking about your concerns, we hope you are able to set aside the time with your partner to identify and talk about a few issues together. Even if you begin by writing notes to one another, it's a good place to start. We can't promise there won't be bumps in the road, but your relationship should grow stronger and healthier with open and respectful communication. Soon, you and your lover can become more comfortable discussing what you both need from your love life after cancer treatment. Then the two of you can begin to experience "great sex" as you've defined it together!

FACT OR FICTION?

"Cancer increases the rate of divorce."

FICTION! There is no evidence that cancer increases the rate of divorce. In fact, for many couples, a crisis such as cancer can make a relationship stronger.

---

[1] Schover LR (1997). Sexuality and Fertility After Cancer, pp. 30-41. New York: John Wiley & Sons, Inc. Reprinted with permission of John Wiley & Sons, Inc.

[2] Tannen D (2001). You Just Don't Understand: Women and Men in Conversation. New York: Harper Paperbacks.

NINE

Sex and the Single Woman

I realized that, as a single woman, I faced a greater emotional risk as I strived to reestablish my life after breast cancer. After all, the question "How do I make love with a man?" isn't clearly asked or answered in the medical literature. And I wanted to know how I would tell a total stranger, not my husband of twenty years, "Yes, I have had breast cancer and had my breast removed. And by the way, I think you are cute."

Linda Dackman, Author
Up Front: Sex and the Post-Mastectomy Woman

We all want to be loved and accepted for who we are, regardless of our imperfections (we all have them). It can be difficult to reveal yourself emotionally and physically to a trusted mate after cancer, but what about to a new lover? How do you talk about it? Who and when do you tell?

Some of you were single during diagnosis and treatment. Others may have been in a long-term relationship that recently ended and find yourselves back on the singles scene. Either way, a common concern is rejection from a potential new partner because of his concern about the possible lingering effects of cancer. Deciding when and with whom to make love after cancer is important. Knowing how and when to tell can make all the difference when you're feeling vulnerable and trying to foster a future romance.

It's really important as a single woman to surround yourself with caring external support. What supportive resources are available to you? Not just for sexual love but also for the unconditional emotional support you deserve during and after cancer treatment. We all need encouragement, to touch and feel connected to others. When we're single, it may be even more essential for us to actively seek out family, friends, support groups, and other resources.

Everything you've read up until now applies to you regardless of whether you are married or single. Each of us must tackle existing body image and self-esteem issues, physical and psychological problems and solutions, and communication challenges after cancer treatment. However, communicating with a new partner is a unique challenge for the single woman. Whether you consider it a benefit or a burden, you have complete control over exactly when and how that conversation should begin.

First and foremost, healthy self-confidence may be the cornerstone of honest communication with a potential new lover. Before you actively pursue dating, ask yourself if you have a clear picture of who you are now. Do you value this woman you see in the mirror? Are you proud of yourself for the strength and courage you have shown? Do you understand that you are much more than a cancer diagnosis or a missing breast?

Cancer happens to all kinds of people, and we can't let a diagnosis define who we are.

Some women seem to believe they're wearing a sign that reads, "I've had cancer." They feel judged by having had cancer and anticipate others' view of them to be based on their diagnosis, as if they were wearing a Scarlet Letter. But think about it. If we were all required to wear scarlet letters identifying our secret sins, no one would be labeled with "C" for cancer. That letter would be saved for those who are cruel, callous, cold-blooded, or cunning. Cancer is not a sin, and you did nothing wrong to get it. You didn't ask to have cancer, nor did you deserve it.

Cancer happens to all kinds of people, and we can't let a diagnosis define who we are. It's important to see beyond the cancer that invaded your life when introducing yourself back into the world. Each of us who has overcome cancer is delighted to be a survivor, but we are more than just survivors, much more than a diagnosis. We are leaders of Brownie packs, ministers, researchers, pilots, quilters – the list goes on. Be confident that you are a beloved, worthy woman with many talents and gifts to offer a new relationship. If you don't truly understand this, perhaps you'll want to sort out your feelings before embarking on a new relationship. When you begin to realize, "He'll be lucky to have me," it might be time to resume dating. The key is to look inward for your value, not outward.

When you are ready to talk about your battle with cancer, more than likely, your potential new love interest will take the cue from you on how to respond to the news. Getting to know this person first will help you decide whether he is worthy of hearing this personal information.

NOT BY CHOICE...

If your former partner or husband left you after you were diagnosed, try to keep these wise words in mind as you accept your new single status:

> *The first husband doesn't want the change; the second husband accepts you as you are.*
>
> *Marsha Kooken, R.N.*

Marsha explains that some men can't handle the changes that cancer brings. For example, some men are clearly "breast men." They are unable to accept that their wives have lost their breasts or had other significant changes to their bodies after cancer. These men end up divorcing their wives, leaving the women to fight the disease and all its lingering effects on their own. Even though getting through the divorce while battling cancer was incredibly difficult, Marsha says a woman is far better off in the long run after this kind of man leaves the relationship. Ultimately, these women end up finding much *better* partners who are aware of the physical changes from the cancer yet desire the women anyway. These are good men, and the women end up more fulfilled and happy with their lives.

BY CHOICE...

Some women reveal they find clarity after a cancer diagnosis. Cancer actually empowers them to leave a bad or unhappy marriage or relationship. Sometimes the relationship wasn't exactly bad, but simply unfulfilling. Regardless, if you find yourself single by choice, you may have fewer issues with self-confidence as you set off on your new solo journey.

> *Jane was shopping and spotted an elderly Nez Perce woman selling jewelry. Jane had a bottle of her husband's favorite wine in a brown paper bag under her arm. After they struck up a conversation, the Nez Perce woman asked, "What's in the bag?" Jane told her, "It's a bottle of wine. I got it for my husband." The Nez Perce woman looked Jane in the eye and said, "Good trade."*
>
> *(Widespread urban legend and Internet joke)*

If you left your partner by choice because you wanted more from your life, now is the time to go and get it. There are, however, still the questions of what, when, and how to tell a new lover about your cancer treatment and its lasting affects.

DON'T CAST YOUR PEARLS BEFORE SWINE...
Who, When, and How To Tell

The Who

In this instance, *you* are the pearl. The message is that you are too precious to hand over your story and yourself to anyone who might not fully appreciate you. However, putting yourself back out there means taking a risk and being vulnerable. When you begin dating, how do you know if you're about to tell your experience to a "swine" or a "keeper"?

> *When I first began telling men about my cancer, I think I "dared" them to reject me. I blurted out, "I've had cancer and am missing a breast" within minutes or hours after our first meeting. I told myself I wanted to know up front whether they could accept me or not. But really, I think I hoped to frighten them away so I didn't have to deal with getting attached and then rejected later.*
>
> Sami*, 37

Sharing significant personal information with a potential new love interest is something like the swift cutting motion of a sharp sword. It separates the "men" from the "boys." Any partner worth having will accept you as you are. Repeat that phrase out loud. "Any partner worth having will accept me as I am." Keep saying it until you truly believe it. It's the absolute truth, and you must feel confident about this fact as you search for a new lover.

Once you have set your sights on someone interesting, get to know this new person. Become friends before you become lovers. When you think you might be ready to share your cancer experience with this person, ask yourself, "Is this someone to whom I would tell my checking account balance?" While some women choose to share their cancer story right from the start, you may be far less vulnerable if you wait until you get to know the person a little more. You might learn about events in his life that could color his reaction to your news. Waiting might help protect you from avoidable hurts. Sharing personal, intimate information with every person you meet is not necessarily empowering.

For instance, if a person has already experienced a loss due to cancer, he may not be capable of having a relationship with you. This doesn't make him a swine; it just means he is not capable of dealing with it. Try not to blame these partners if a relationship with you is going to be too difficult for them. Let them go without anger. In the end, creating a healthy relationship might have been too difficult for both of you.

Some prospective partners may not know how to react when you tell them about your cancer, but it will not keep them from pursuing you. True, some will not be interested in dating you once told about your cancer diagnosis. Just remember that the cutting sword of truth helps you sort the swine from the keepers. It is better to know whether or not a potential partner can accept this part of you before investing too much of yourself in the relationship. Still, the question remains, when is the right time to tell a new potential love interest about your personal journey?

The When

In Dr. Kydd's workshops on intimacy after cancer, a number of single women who overcame breast cancer shared their stories about telling a new lover about the cancer. Each woman told the new lover just before they were going to make love. The same disastrous result happened every time; there was no lovemaking and the guys left without returning. Don't repeat their mistakes!

> *I told him about my missing breast as he was taking off my shirt in the heat of passion. He stopped and said, "what?" He seemed stunned and told me he couldn't handle it right now. He left. I thought we had something good together, so now I'm confused and a little devastated. After all, I'm a strong, vibrant woman who has just overcome a life-threatening illness. What has he done lately?*
>
> *Katy*, 35

Several women who waited to tell had similar outcomes. They dated a guy a few times; then as things suddenly turned sexual and they were pulling each other's clothes off, the women blurted out their news about cancer and missing breasts or scars. Each time, the words jolted the guy from accelerating desire to an icy halt. Some of the men were swine – not worthy of these women. Some were simply stunned into silence, wondering why the women hadn't told them before this. Things may go better if you pick a time to talk about your cancer deliberately; the throes of passion is probably not the best time.

When do you tell a potential new lover about your cancer and the changes to your body? Some women choose to mention it at a first meeting. In most cases, this may be "too much information" up front. How would you respond if someone you just met said something like, "Hi, my name is John, and I had an alcoholic father who beat me regularly?" First, you might wonder, "Why is he telling me this? I hardly know him!" Or perhaps you would have a lot of questions about his statement but wonder if asking them is appropriate. You might even wonder what baggage he carried from this critical life event. It is not a normal way to find out personal information about someone you just met. Neither is, "Hi, my name is Betty, and I am missing a breast due to breast cancer."

> *The best time to bring up your cancer experience is probably when you are both discussing your personal life stories.*

A more appropriate first step is to get to know the person. Become friends. Talk about ordinary things. Enjoy what couples on normal dates enjoy before they are intimate. You may know after the first three or four dates whether or not you like this person enough to continue dating or decide he is really not your type. If you decide the latter, then you haven't divulged any deeply personal information. If you do want to continue dating, then you can decide when the time is right to talk about your medical history.

While each relationship is unique, the best time to bring up your cancer experience is probably when you are both discussing your personal life stories, such as whether either of you has been married before, has children, still wants or can have children, or the fulfilled dreams and tragedies of your lives. In the normal course of more intimate conversation, it is appropriate to bring up your own courageous story about cancer.

THE HOW

> *One thing that's not discussed is being single...there should be more education on how to get past that, to get yourself-esteem because to be honest, it's not easy being single, especially if you've had a mastectomy, when you don't feel whole, and that's a big issue to be able to go on in life and feel that you can be with a partner and feel sexy and desirable.*
>
> *Anonymous, (Toronto)*
> *In <u>Nothing Fit Me: The information and Support Needs of Canadian Young Women with Breast Cancer,</u> CBCN Final Report, January 2003*

If you're wondering *how* to tell a future lover about the changes to your body since cancer, remember you are not alone. Many women wonder how to delicately bring this knowledge into a new relationship. It might help to consider how common cancer really is in our society. Each of us knows someone who has had cancer. Cancer doesn't make you a freak of nature. It may have made you a stronger woman, though.

Once you've decided on the "who" and the "when," it is time to tackle the "how" of telling. It's probably best to keep this conversation out of the bedroom. Try scheduling a time for uninterrupted talk, or simply decide you are going to broach the subject at your next date, especially if the date will be just the two of you at a quiet location. The point is to discuss the subject only when you've consciously decided the time is right for you. If you are worried about what you will say, write the words down and practice saying them to yourself or to a trusted friend until they roll off your lips easily.

Be honest. Talk slowly and deliberately. Don't rush through your story, but keep it brief and to the point. Just tell the basics about your diagnosis and treatment. If you are missing a breast(s) or have had reconstructive surgery, say so. Describe your scars. In essence, prepare this person to see you naked. Give this potential new lover a few minutes to digest what you are saying. Remember, we all have scars, whether or not they show.

Be open to questions. Your new partner may be stunned, frightened, or just trying to think of how to reassure you that he accepts this part of you. Give him a few minutes. Remember, men don't multi-task as women do; they quickly fire up the problem-solving part of their brain when faced with a dilemma.

When you've both had a chance to talk about it for as long as needed, perhaps the two of you can agree to talk about it again later if the new partner has any concerns.

Be prepared – your potential new partner may respond with something other than support. Having this conversation may end your budding relationship. However, you were in control of both the timing and the content of the conversation, and you did it with your clothes on. Rejection in the heat of passion while you're both getting naked and vulnerable could have been far worse.

It's also quite possible that this person will respond to your cancer experience with strength, compassion, and tenderness. Many women who have found joy in the support of a new love interest describe how this initial conversation about their cancer experience made them feel closer to their new lover. Whether or not this new love interest becomes a life partner, taking the risk with someone who interests you is almost always worth it.

> *We met at a mutual friends' house and casually had dinner together two times. When he asked me out for a third time, I answered, "First, I think you should know I've had breast cancer and am missing a breast." He said, "So that prevents you from eating?" We had dinner and a lot more that night and are still together two years later.*
>
> *Clairese*, 48*

NOW THAT YOU KNOW BETTER...

Your cancer journey has been an exceptionally important part of your life, or perhaps *the* most significant thing that has ever happened to you. Treat it like any other momentous personal life event. Guard your heart, and yet at the same time, be willing to put yourself back out into the world. You have to take the risk of trusting another person to reap the benefits of developing a romantic and sexual relationship. Only you will know when you are ready; but don't forget, sometimes we have to seize an opportunity even though it scares us.

When the time is right for making love to a new partner, apply all that you learned in previous chapters to your sexual encounter. For instance, wear a camisole or lingerie during lovemaking if it makes you more confident. Some women say they feel sexy wearing just their partner's white button-down cotton shirt, leaving only the center button clasped. Remember, before you begin to make love, talk with your partner about any limitations you may have, such as needing lubrication and having to position yourself on top to succeed. Most importantly, don't forget the lubrication and your sense of humor!

The choice of when, how, and with whom to share your cancer journey is entirely your choice to make. If you want a potential partner to know about it up front, you have every right to share it. However, try to understand that sharing too much information with virtual strangers may be a little scary to some would-be partners. Besides, you might want to discern the swine from the keeper first and decide whether the person you are telling is worthy of knowing this much about you.

SINGLES NEED SEXUAL SUPPORT, TOO!

My oncologist told me he wasn't sure why I kept asking about sexual side effects of my cancer treatment. He said since I didn't have a partner, it really shouldn't matter.

Dawn*, 55

It is imperative that you seek treatment for any sexual side effects, such as menopausal symptoms, that result from cancer and its treatment. Do not feel ashamed to ask for help, whether you are single *or* married. This is not the Dark Ages. It's important to treat the very real and sometimes long-lasting physical side effects of cancer treatment early on. If a health professional responds with indifference, then get another opinion. There are excellent, knowledgeable professionals available to treat your symptoms without question. It doesn't matter that you don't have a life partner. Your sexual issues still need to be addressed.

Everything you read in Chapter Four about menopausal symptoms of dry vagina, thin vaginal walls, and narrowing vaginal opening pertains to you. These are uncomfortable symptoms that need treatment. Lubricants and vaginal moisturizers can help relieve some symptoms. Also, just because you don't have a partner to experiment with doesn't mean you shouldn't figure out what works and what feels good on your own. If you ignore these symptoms, you may not be able to function fully when you do find a lover.

If you have not yet begun dating, remember that self-stimulation is a good way to explore your new sexual capacity after cancer treatment. Self-stimulation can also soothe sexual frustrations. Most importantly, it will help maintain the tone and elasticity of your vagina after cancer treatment (see Chapter Seven for more information). Remember: If you don't use it, you'll lose it.

WHERE TO FIND DATES AFTER TREATMENT

Dating is challenging even when you haven't had cancer. How do you get back out into the dating scene after cancer? The answer is fairly simple, at least it's simple to say: Open yourself up to new friendships and new lovers.

It's important to be realistic in setting standards when selecting a new lover. No one can meet every one of our expectations or hopes, so try to prioritize the truly important characteristics of your new mate. If you're not really sure what you want, try making a list of qualities or characteristics you'd like to see in a partner.

When you are ready to date, tell your friends, family, co-workers, and neighbors. Many people have found true love through mutual acquaintances. Coffee shops, bookstores, churches, synagogues, volunteering and political events are all good places to meet other singles. You might consider developing a new interest, attempting a new hobby, or taking a class at your local college or community center. You could even get a dog and walk through the dog parks to meet other pet owners. The important thing is to get out of your comfort zone and just do it!

Some women choose to ask an old lover or a close friend to be their first sexual contact after cancer treatment. The level of trust they feel with a past lover or friend allows them to be more at ease when "testing the waters". If you decide to ask a previous partner or friend to be your "first" after treatment, make it clear that you do not intend for this to be a long-term relationship, just a way to jump start your sex life with someone you trust.

On the other hand, if you've experienced many failed relationships or have tended to go for the wrong kind of guy in the past, this may be a great time for you to take an honest look at yourself. Figure out why previous relationships ended and decide what you want from a future relationship. You may do this assessment on your own or seek professional counseling. Once you determine what you truly want from a future relationship, we hope you go after it with a zest for life and find exactly what you are looking for!

KEEP IT SAFE, SISTER

Even if you think you can't get pregnant after treatment, it is extremely important to practice safe sex. Use a condom. Slather it with a lubricant if you need to, and be sure to only use a lubricant that won't destroy the condom (see Chapter Five for more detailed information).

An unwanted pregnancy may not be the only outcome of unprotected sex. Many newly single women develop infections from sexually transmitted diseases, including hepatitis or HIV/AIDS; they may have been afraid to ask their new partner(s) about their sexual history or just haven't had to think about safe sex until now. Even if you are post-menopausal or can no longer have children, having safe sex is vital to your health. When you've had chemotherapy, your immune system weakens, making you more susceptible to infections; this is particularly true if you've had a blood cancer or a bone marrow transplant. No matter who you choose to become intimate with, insist on using a condom.

WE ALL NEED LOVE

During and after a life-changing event like cancer, we each need to know that our life matters, and that we are loved. We need hugs, touches, kisses, and a caring soul to listen to us. If you are single, you must find that valuable support in places other than a life partner. The good news is that there are many resources available to help you find effective and loving support. You can find encouragement and assistance through trusted friends, extended family members, and close colleagues or co-workers. You can also seek help from your spiritual advisor, people involved in your religious organization, or through volunteer and community connections you've made.

Another wonderful place to find the support you need is through the many cancer care organizations that exist. Go online and search for programs through the American Cancer Society, the Canadian Breast Care Network (CBCN), and other support organizations such as Gilda's Club or Reach to Recovery to locate the support you need and deserve. These organizations will put you in touch with other women who have gone through similar life-altering experiences. For more information, refer to the Resources section at the end of this book.

The issue for some women, however, is *not* that they do not have resources but that they are often afraid to ask for help. This is no time to be shy or proud. Once you open up to others, you may be pleased to discover just how caring other people can be when they are needed.

FACT OR FICTION?

"Once you are no longer fertile, you don't need to use contraceptives."

FICTION! In truth, your body may be more susceptible to infection and sexually transmitted diseases after cancer treatment, such as chemotherapy. You may also still risk becoming pregnant. Practicing safe sex after cancer treatment is vital.

Ten

It's Not About Me When...

No one can make you feel inferior without your permission.

Eleanor Roosevelt

W omen too often look inward and blame themselves when things go wrong. For instance, when our families are in crisis or when there are problems at work, we look inside ourselves and ask, "What mistake did I make for this to happen?" or "How can I do things differently so this doesn't happen again?" We may even ask ourselves, "What can I learn from this?"

Men certainly don't sit around with friends discussing their expanding bottoms and whether or not they look good naked. If they do mention weight, some will laugh it off while they pat their beer bellies. Men don't usually agonize about their appearance or stop living a full life because they think their bodies aren't perfect. They also don't blame themselves for an insensitive comment someone else makes to them. So how come women do?

As women, when a person says something insensitive or unkind to us, we often accept and internalize those thoughtless words. We blame ourselves for imperfections. Even when we don't agree with the hurtful words, we spend a lot of energy wondering, "Why would she say something like that to me?" This may be one of the few times it would be better to think like a man! Instead of absorbing those inconsiderate words, we need to deflect them and understand the problem lies with the person who said them. We must learn to place external blame versus internal blame from impolite, insensitive comments.

THINKING LIKE A MAN...NO PERSONALIZATION!

Remember in Chapter Three when we discussed the power of your thoughts and common "cognitive distortions?" Do you recall the cognitive distortion entitled "Personalization?" It's when you blame yourself for something terrible or insensitive that another person says or does. You may think you caused the negative external event when, in fact, you are not responsible for it.

When you have cancer, you face many difficulties, most of which are out of your control. You are not responsible for the cancer, nor are you responsible for the way it might have changed your body and mind. You can, however, choose to overcome the hurdles you face after cancer. You also have the power to *not* let other people's thoughtless comments affect you. You don't have to "own" their insensitive remarks. Try to think like a man in this instance...know that the problem lies within the person making the remarks and has nothing to do with you.

What lies behind us, and what lies before us are tiny matters compared to what lies within us.

Ralph Waldo Emerson

EXTERNAL PERSONALITY GROUPS

The list of insensitive remarks said to people in crisis is endless. Part of the problem is that, sometimes, you have to go through the crisis to truly understand how it feels. If a person hasn't had cancer, he or she can't completely understand your experience. Even when the other person had cancer, our own experiences are nevertheless unique.

A compassionate, caring person may still unintentionally say the wrong thing simply because he or she doesn't know it is insensitive. Their intent may be good, but their words careless. When you respond to their comments, try to keep in mind their good intentions toward you.

Another type of insensitivity lies with the person who doesn't know what to say. This person is nervous to talk about your illness and probably has a difficult time addressing intense or emotional issues in general. Their blunders are not meant to hurt you. This uneasy person simply doesn't know any better, although perhaps they need to be educated.

The third type of insensitive talk comes from the person who really doesn't want to be bothered with things that don't affect him or her, and that includes your cancer. They know they *should* say something, but it takes too much effort for them to think of a suitable thing to say. They want to hurry and "get it out of the way" so they can go on to "more important tasks" that usually involve them. Again, the problem lies within this selfish person and has nothing to do with you. If you want, you can take this person to task when appropriate.

TLC – TOTALLY LUDICROUS COMMENTS?

The following are examples of the kinds of insensitive comments that are frequently spoken to people who've had cancer. We hope they will help you see that the comments are not about you personally. The remarks say more about the other person, who is undoubtedly insensitive or simply uninformed.

It's Not About Me When...
My doctor is uncomfortable talking
about my sexual problems.

This may be a good example of someone who is normally a compassionate person who is saying the wrong thing. Many health professionals, such as doctors, are not comfortable talking about sexual issues. This is *their problem,* not yours! You have a right and a personal responsibility to ask about your sexual health.

Just when you have gotten up the courage to ask your doctor about the sexual issues you're having since treatment, you might come across a doctor who is either too busy or is equally if not more embarrassed talking about sex than you. Thankfully, many doctors and other health professionals are wonderful and very comfortable talking about this topic. It may help to try to remember they are human beings too and are not immune from feeling awkward about the subject. However, if you get a response that does not answer your questions about your sexual side effects, then ask if there is someone else you can talk with about these issues. Don't let one uncomfortable conversation prevent you from seeking the help you need to live a full, satisfying life.

It's Not About Me When...
Your partner no longer appears
interested in you sexually.

Your partner could be the one with the decreased libido. It's possible your lover still sees you as fragile or unhealthy. If your partner sees you as an invalid and is afraid of hurting you, he or she is not going to be thinking about having sex with you.

The most important step in resolving this issue is communication. Remember, this isn't about you; it is about your partner's fears. Talk about your concerns together. Even if your partner remains uninterested in sex, at least you will know where you stand in your future relationship with him or her. If neither of you communicates your concerns, then it *does* become your problem.

If your partner says he or she is afraid of or turned off by your new body (which is hardly ever the case), the two of you can talk about it. Remember, this is *still* about your partner and not you, even though it is about your body. Other partners have no trouble accepting their lover's new body after cancer; this is your partner's problem, not yours. By talking about it, the two of you can find ways to deal with it. For instance, you can wear special lingerie (discussed in Chapter Seven) or teach him or her how to focus on other sensual parts of your body. Develop an entirely new sexual script, which may help invigorate your old sex life. However, you will never get to this place if the two of you don't communicate your concerns to each other.

If both of you are no longer interested in sex, it is still worth talking about. You can eliminate any guilt either of you may be feeling about it. Then the two of you can feel intimate or connected to one another even if you are not sexually active.

IT'S NOT ABOUT ME WHEN...
PEOPLE MAKE THOUGHTLESS COMMENTS, SUCH AS, "I
KNOW HOW YOU FEEL," OR, "YOU DON'T LOOK SICK,"
OR, "AT LEAST THE CANCER WASN'T THAT BAD," OR,
"WELL THAT'S OVER AND DONE WITH NOW."

The list of foolish, thoughtless comments spoken to people in a crisis such as cancer is unfortunately very long. No doubt, you have probably been told by an acquaintance that you "look great!" This is not exactly what you want to hear when you are terrified and in for the fight of your life.

Dr. Kydd wears her hair short. At the time of her cancer diagnosis, she was in the process of buying a house and was meeting with a realtor. Dr. Kydd mentioned to the realtor one day that she was surprised to find herself more concerned about losing her hair from chemotherapy than about the major surgery that awaited. The realtor replied, "I can't imagine why you are concerned about losing your hair when you have so little of it to begin with!"

A woman at one of Dr. Kydd's intimacy after cancer workshops said an acquaintance had asked, "So which tit did you lose?" We know each of you has a similar story to tell. Tales of inappropriate comments abound. These insensitive people speak volumes about their lack of empathy, their fear about cancer, and their selfishness. *It is NOT about you.* It's just unfortunate that you have to deal with these comments when what you could really benefit from is some TLC – "Tender Loving Care," rather than TLC – "Totally Ludicrous Comments."

It's Not About Me When...
People avoid me at work, at the supermarket, and at social events.

Frequently, people are clueless about what to say and what not to say in response to a crisis such as cancer. This may be especially true if they have not experienced tragedy in their own lives, because they don't know how to relate to it. Quite often, people are scared that they could even "catch" cancer. Remember that when they avoid you, it is their problem, not yours. They may have no experience with critical life events and are, therefore, clumsy when responding to yours. The bottom line is that they are avoiding their own fears and inadequacies, and not you.

In life, there is a saying that there are good experiences, and there are learning experiences...cancer is definitely a learning experience. You learn an awful lot about other people – which people are kind, caring, and want to help. You also learn about those who are uncomfortable with the situation, those who are not used to being around sickness, or those who have never had to deal with difficult issues before. You learn quickly to distinguish people of compassion, those who are there for *you,* from those who would rather run and hide. Place the inconsiderate behavior back on them; *it is not about you.* Learn about the true person through their behavior in a time of need. The weakness lies in them.

It's Not About Me When...
My partner leaves me after I'm
diagnosed with cancer.

It may at first feel like another huge loss at a time when you're dealing with more than you could ever have imagined. Marriage vows of "in sickness and in health" fall by the wayside. Those vows were written deliberately because no one wants a "fair weather" partner. Life gets messy. None of us is immune from hardships or disease such as cancer. It could have happened to your partner. Would you have left him or her because of it? Again, it speaks volumes about the weakness and flaws in the other person, *not you.*

It doesn't matter whether you are married or not; what matters is whether or not the person you are with is trying to ease your burden. Going through a break up after cancer treatment doesn't feel like a good thing. However, if a partner leaves you because you got cancer, you are truly better off in the long run, though it might not feel like it at the time.

Sometimes *it is about you.* For some women, a cancer diagnosis helps them realize they've been in an unfulfilling or harmful relationship. Now that they've been given a second chance at life, they don't want to waste a minute of it. If a cancer diagnosis helps you comprehend that your intimate relationship hasn't added any value to your life, you may choose to end it. In this case, it is about you making a powerful, thoughtful decision to improve your life.

It's Not About Me When...
I lose my hair with chemotherapy.

You have no control over whether your hair falls out from chemotherapy. You didn't ask for cancer, nor did you deserve to lose your hair.

However, *it is about you* if you lose your self-esteem because of it. Chemotherapy causes drastic physical changes while it attacks and removes cancer cells from your body. That's its job. Sure, you may feel exhausted or changed, but you are a very special person who is enduring huge physical changes in the process of getting healthy again. Review the chapter on self-esteem if needed; having a healthy sense of yourself is vital. It's okay to lose your hair, but don't lose your hope or your self-esteem.

It's Not About Me When…
My family isn't helpful.

It *is about you* if you let this continue. Previously, you may have been Superwoman; being and doing all things for those you love. Your family benefited from your super human strength, skills, and competency. Yet now, all of those female multi-tasking super human powers must concentrate on making you well again. There isn't much energy left to care for your family right now. All the same, your family members are capable of caring for themselves, especially in your time of need – that is, if you'll let them.

Try talking with your family to let them know that things have to be different. Tell them they ought to do extra work so you can get the rest you need while you recover. This holds true even after treatments have stopped. Your body is still working hard to heal.

If your family is not responsive to your requests for sharing the load, remember *it is not about you. It is about them.* The only way to reconcile this situation is for you to decide you will not attempt to do it all for them; your family needs to step up to the plate and work together for you and for the good of the entire family.

It's Not About Me When…
I have physical side effects from cancer treatment such as vaginal dryness.

It *is about you* if you do nothing to resolve your side effects from treatment. We hope we have been able to provide you with ideas on how to deal with these side effects, including seeking treatment from your health professional.

Don't let the physical side effects from cancer treatment stop you from having a fulfilling intimate relationship. Get the Replens, buy the lubrication, use the vibrator if necessary, speak to your gynecologist, and seek out the help you need to overcome any sexual difficulties. It will be worth the effort!

It's Not About Me When...
I get upset about my diagnosis.

A cancer diagnosis can be incredibly isolating, and *it is not about you* when you feel upset by it. It *is about you* if you just give in, or don't eventually rally to decide that hope is more important than despair. It is understandable if you feel depressed with your situation; who wouldn't? But if you have lost all hope, it may be time to seek help from a professional counselor. In addition, you can join a support group or a dragon boat team, or get together with other women who have "been there, done that" who can help you move forward on the road ahead.

It's Not About Me When...
Well, maybe it is about me if I get upset by well-meaning, well-intentioned comments.

Many people don't know what to say after a person has had cancer. A frequent comment made by some very well-meaning people is, "Oh, you look well," as if they expect you to look ill forever. Of course, we'd rather hear that we look great than, "Oh, you look terrible," but it can be upsetting if you remember that they never commented about your appearance prior to your illness. They are inadvertently defining you by your cancer.

The truth is, any well-meaning comment can be misunderstood and misconstrued, especially when we feel self-conscious or are experiencing low self-esteem. Dr. Kydd says she always feels like responding to the "You look great" comment with, "Well, I looked my best the day before my diagnosis when I still had cancer." It *is about you* if you let well-intended comments like this one get to you.

GOODNESS IS ABOUT YOU!

Most importantly, do not be discouraged by insensitive people or their comments. No one knows how you feel except you, and your feelings are completely valid. Remember, *it is about them, not you.*

When you encounter upsetting, thoughtless remarks, stop and question why it is happening. Try to realize the ownership for the unhelpful comments lies with the person speaking and not you. When such situations arise, we challenge you to come up with your own versions of "It's Not About Me When..."

We all know that at the end of the day, *it IS about you!* Seek out the positive influences and try to let go of the negative ones. Be glad that people care enough and are brave enough to ask how you are or to comment about your health.

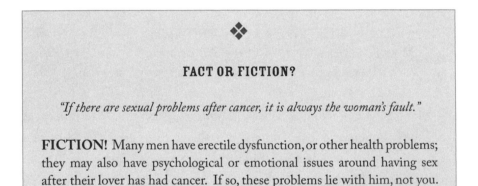

FACT OR FICTION?

"If there are sexual problems after cancer, it is always the woman's fault."

FICTION! Many men have erectile dysfunction, or other health problems; they may also have psychological or emotional issues around having sex after their lover has had cancer. If so, these problems lie with him, not you. It's not your fault.

Eleven

For Husbands and Partners

NOTE

This chapter is written for your husband or partner. It will briefly explain your side effects since treatment, and identify the kind of support you need.

My wife is a wonder. She wonders where to shop every day.

You might be wondering why your wife or partner handed you a chapter in the book she's been reading. It's because this chapter was written specifically for you. She is having ongoing side effects from her cancer treatment. To make matters worse, these side effects are difficult to talk about. In a nutshell, she's concerned about the way you view her since cancer, the way she views herself, and her ability to enjoy intimacy with you now. None of these issues is easy to discuss, even if you've been together for a long time. However, if you do make the effort to talk about them, your intimate relationship may vastly improve.

You've both been through a great deal since her diagnosis and treatment. Life *after* cancer can also be challenging. You may be wondering, "When can life get back to normal or be about something other than cancer?" The good news is that cancer and its lingering effects don't have to dominate your lives. She wants a more normal life and knows you do too; the only dilemma is that your "normal life" has probably changed.

Marc Silver, in his book <u>Breast Cancer Husband</u>, explains that the "old normal," or your life before cancer, has changed; you now have a "new normal," which is your life after cancer.[1] You might as well know that you can't return to the old normal or the way life was before cancer. This fact can be upsetting to both of you. She is acutely aware of this reality and is possibly grieving the loss of her old self right now; maybe you are too. This doesn't mean that either of you has to throw out your previous passions or way of life; it's just that they might need some tweaking.

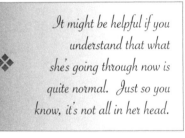

It might be helpful if you understand that what she's going through now is quite normal. Just so you know, it's not all in her head.

One of the things that a cancer diagnosis can do is make you both take a good look at your lives. Once you've made it through the crisis of her diagnosis and treatment, you are not the same people as when you started. No one survives cancer and remains the same. She might be stronger, quieter, louder, softer, angrier, happier, or more withdrawn than she was before; the same holds true for you. Her body also changes with treatment. Of course, the most important thing is to get rid of the cancer...but then what? What are the two of you left with?

Treatment was no doubt difficult. She may have lost breast(s) or other body parts from surgery, and possibly gone through the rigors of chemotherapy or radiation. But did you know that the side effects of cancer treatment last long after treatment has stopped? Just when you think it's over and you can "get back to normal," you both discover changes to her body. Besides being surgically scarred, she may have symptoms such as hot flashes, night sweats, or trouble sleeping. If so, she's likely having additional side effects that she might not have told you about yet.

Then there are the psychological effects of cancer. Cancer is frightening. Now that she's made it past treatment, your partner or wife knows she should be happy that she's alive, and she is. Yet it's not uncommon for grief and depression to come and go or last long after a crisis like cancer has passed.

It might be helpful if you understand that what she's going through now is quite normal. Just so you know, it's not all in her head. She has been left with some very real physical and psychological side effects of treatment. Her body doesn't work the same way as it did, and she's frustrated and saddened by this fact. She might also be looking to you for confirmation that she is still a loved, desirable woman. The confusing part for you is that she might be acting as if this is the *last* thing she wants from you.

The best thing you can do while she is dealing with the after-effects of treatment is to just be there for her. Make her feel that she has a safe environment to express her concerns and reassure her that she is still the same person you've always loved with or without her breasts. This is true even if you really miss her breasts (or any other change to her body). If she can tell you about her physical sexual limitations since treatment, and if she feels accepted and loved just as she is, you'll see the girl you fell in love with. It's possible that your relationship will be even better than it was before cancer.

WOMEN THINK OUT LOUD, AND MEN TAKE ACTION!

When my wife has a problem, she talks about it forever. Sometimes, it drives me nuts.

It's common knowledge that men and women think differently. A woman's brain is programmed to talk through a problem until she reaches a resolution. A man's brain is pre-wired to think problems over silently until he finds a solution. When she "wants to talk about it," she is actually working through a problem and is looking for empathy and a way to feel connected to you. She is probably *not* looking for advice.

Unfortunately for women sometimes, men are solution-oriented. That means you are programmed to either "fix it" or to offer advice on how to fix it. But when you give advice, she interprets this as you not listening to her (what she wants), and she may feel that you are not concerned about the issue. Guess what? *You can't fix it, and she needs to talk about it.* So where does that leave you (brace yourself)…it leaves you…listening.

Most men don't want to hear a lot of words; they want to take action. Even as a man hears the words, "blah blah you blah sex blah blah," a man is thinking about the best solution to the problem. If this sounds like you, you're in good company. *However,* you may need to adjust your thinking on this one. Listening to her *is* fixing the problem. She will eventually arrive at the solution as she talks it through; or maybe *there is no solution.* She may not need answers but only to know that you care about what she is feeling.

If your mate keeps all of her thoughts and heartache bottled up because she is afraid you don't want to hear it, the answers won't come and things might get worse. This is not to say that you have to quietly listen to hours upon hours of talking. She's already read about having a time limit when expressing one or two important issues with you. You'll have a chance to respond and convey your own concerns. You can both agree on how best to communicate the issues that she is facing since treatment. The important part is to start talking and actively listening. Here's an example of how you can "fix it" by listening.

> **She:** *"I am unhappy with my looks. I miss my breast. I hate cancer. I am not sure if I can ever be naked in front of you again; I don't even want to look at my scar. I am alive but I feel so sad and then I feel guilty because I should be happy…"*

> **You:** *(Listening…listening…listening…occasionally nodding so she knows you are listening) Uh huh.*

> **She:** *"…and I'm all mixed up inside." (Silence)*

> **You:** *"I love you. I want you. I need you. You are still a very attractive woman..." or "I love you, and I still want you when you are ready."*

If it applies, you might also say something like,

> **You:** *"I miss your breast too, but I would miss you more," or "Your missing breasts don't matter to me, but I'm trying to support how you feel about it."*

The point is that she needs to hear loudly and clearly that you accept and love her regardless of what cancer has done to her body. You might assume she knows this because you are still there, showing your love and concern. Yet she still needs to hear those words from your lips. You may have to repeat these words many times over the next days, weeks, and months. But it will be worth it. What she doesn't need is for you to dismiss her fears as "silly" or to tell her that she should just drop it and move on.

If you have been holding her hand through surgery, chemotherapy, and doctor appointments, this initial conversation might be easier. Yet for many men, displaying emotional support does not come easily. If your way of showing her support through diagnosis and treatment was to work harder at your job to make sure she was provided for, she might need to hear that now, too. It could be that when she saw you paying more attention to your job, she felt you were ignoring or rejecting her at a crucial time in her life. Her perception of your behavior can lead to resentment that will not make her feel much desire for romance. What you intended as good, she may interpret as hurtful. Open communication is the only way to set it right.

WHEN WORDS SPEAK LOUDER THAN ACTIONS

> *My wife says she needs more affection from me. I don't get it...I just washed her car yesterday!*

When you are silent about your own concerns, she may feel unloved. You may be quietly anxious about having sex with her after she recovers. You might be nervous that you will hurt her. You may be worried that you will push her into something she's not yet ready for. You can probably check this one off of your list. If she's reading this book, she is either ready to resume an active sexual relationship or she is trying to get ready.

While you might be nervous about touching her, she might need you to at least try. It's possible that she will say, "No, I'm not ready yet." So what? The thing is, when you don't try to touch her the way you used to, she may interpret this as you being repulsed or turned off by her appearance.

She may withdraw further or become angry if you don't attempt to touch her. Your response might be to back off still further. This will make her feel even more rejected by you. As you can see, it's a vicious spiral of no sex, compounded by a misunderstanding, no sex, and so on.

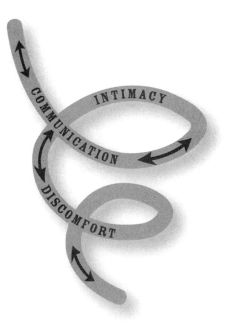

If you want to resume having sexual relations, ask her. You may have to make the first move. Perhaps the best way to find out if she's ready is to say something like, "Tell me how to love you," or "Tell me what you need." Because her body is undergoing many changes, she must feel free to tell you when she wants to try again and what she is capable of doing. If she's not yet ready, then "No" means no. Just so you know, she has learned from previous chapters about other ways for the two of you to enjoy intimacy if she is not yet capable of having intercourse. When she is prepared to discuss it, she can share those ways with you.

The bottom line sexually is that it is vital that you treat her similar to the way you did before cancer. For instance, if you used to playfully pinch at her breasts, she still needs this kind of sexual attention. If her breasts are gone, you can find a new playful sexual tease. Try patting her bottom or stroking her hair to show your desire of her.

If you're worried about hurting her, then just ask her, "Will it hurt if I touch you here?" and, "Do you want me to?" It might also be a good idea to simply ask her what she wants and needs from you. Her body might still be tender from treatment, and she might not want much touching yet. The best way to know what each of you wants is to talk about it.

INTIMACY VERSUS SEX

Intimacy means she might use the word "cuddle" when you're thinking, "I can't wait to get some tonight."

Intimacy isn't necessarily sex. Intimacy is feeling close to one another (yes, it includes cuddling). It can involve sexual touch, such as passionate kissing, stroking, holding, caressing, or lying together with your clothes on or off. It's not a bad place to start. She might need intimacy for a while before she is able to have sex. This means that she needs you to touch her, hug her, and kiss her without expecting it to lead to sex. Foreplay for a woman begins in her mind, and she usually has to feel connected to you emotionally before she wants to get naked with you.

Sex, as you knew it before, might also need to change for a time. If so, there's a reason, and she wants to tell you what it is. Yes, it could be that her interest is low. It could also be that she's nervous that the sexual contact will be painful or impossible due to her current physical symptoms.

SEX AFTER CANCER: JUST THE FACTS, MAN

*Men don't ask for directions and don't read instructions...even
for sex. Just show us the parts, and we'll put it together.*

Cancer treatment can cause severe symptoms of menopause (it doesn't
matter how young she is) and also a reduced interest in sex. It's not her
fault. Cancer treatment can be a passion killer. She's not rejecting you.
She is trying to revive her interest and ability.

Just so you know, cancer treatment can make a woman's vagina really
dry, thin, and narrow (we have to use the "V" word, so prepare yourself if it
makes you uncomfortable). This means it's nearly impossible or extremely
painful to have sexual intercourse or possibly any kind of sexual contact.
Her vagina can tear easily and bleed, and this really hurts! Also, her body
may not heal the same way it would have before cancer.

The mere thought of sex might make her tense up, which of course,
makes it worse. An analogy to help you understand the level of her
discomfort: A woman trying to have sexual contact with a dry, thin,
and narrow vagina is similar to a man rubbing sand paper on an erect
penis. Ouch! Where is the pleasure in that? You can understand why
her desire for this kind of contact is slim to nil. The good news is that
there are many ways to enhance her ability to enjoy sex again. And the
great news is that she wants to! You may have to be patient and open
to a little sexual exploration while you both figure it out.

What does this mean? Will she ever enjoy sex again? For now, it
simply means that the two of you need to talk about what you both need
and want from your intimate relationship. Do you want sex yet? Do you
need sex every day? Perhaps your desire has been reduced too, and you're
okay with waiting. If so, make sure she knows your lack of desire is not
because you're repulsed by her new body but because you want to wait until
it's right for both of you. You might also still see her as a person who is ill
and not yet think of her as a sexual being again. If that's the case, it's time
to start thinking of her as a desirable woman again. She's ready...mostly.

You can feel confident that she is working on ways to enjoy having sex with you again. Her current physical changes don't mean that she will never be able to enjoy sex. You both can! It just means that you might have to try some different ways than what you were used to before cancer. For example, using safe, appropriate lubricants and trying new positions can really help. Also know that wild, passionate lovemaking may be out of the question for now.

This is part of what she wants to discuss with you. But as you can see, it's not an easy subject to bring up. Hopefully, we'll give you enough information so that you both feel more comfortable when discussing this subject.

If sexual intercourse is not possible for now, it might help to know there are many other ways to enjoy one another sexually. If you haven't been open to other ways of making love, you might want to give it some serious thought. We're not talking kinky sex, just trying out some new things. There is no right or wrong answer to how you feel close to one another; it's a matter of personal choice. No one gets to decide this but the two of you, and she must lead this experimentation by telling you what she wants to try and what she is capable of trying.

PLAYING SOLITAIRE...

Sex is like playing cards. Sometimes you have to play by yourself until your partner arrives.

Self-stimulation is an option for you until your wife or partner is able to join you. Some men need to have sex often, and that doesn't change just because their mate is unable to join in. If you are one of these men, self-stimulation may help reduce sexual frustration. Also, your wife or partner may be willing and able to stimulate you until she can participate. It's something you should talk about together so she doesn't misinterpret what you are doing alone as further rejection of her.

When the two of you begin to explore, know that a lubricant is needed no matter how you touch her sexually below the waist. A lubricant should be placed on anything that you intend to use to touch her, including your fingers. This helps reduce the risk of tearing her vagina or causing her pain and discomfort.

While you are playing solitaire, you should know that she has been informed about trying this on herself. There are several good reasons for her to try self-stimulation. First, she needs to explore her new body to see what feels good now and what doesn't; you see, what worked for her before cancer may not feel good after treatment. Once she figures out what works, she can share that information with you. If you try to satisfy her sexually before she understands her own body after cancer, you could unintentionally hurt her. It could also be embarrassing for both of you if you are trying to tenderly touch her, and she is yelling "ouch!"

Also, think about introducing sex toys and fantasy into your relationship. These can be great ways to reinvigorate a "quiet" sex life. However, *safety is key!* She'll have to be careful not to use anything that will cause harm to her vulnerable, tender body. But if you've never looked at these items together before, they can be a fun way to reintroduce sex and humor into your relationship. See, we told you that your "new normal" might be better than ever.

If either of you have religious or other beliefs that prevent you from self-stimulation, there are still other methods to help you return to a satisfying sexual relationship. Once the two of you begin to talk about it, she can let you know what those methods are, or you can read about them in Chapter Seven of this book.

BRING YOUR SENSE OF HUMOR...

After surgery, I had two different sized breasts. I was concerned about my husband's reaction to my lopsided body. He looked at me lovingly and said, "It's great! It's like being with two different women at the same time!" We both laughed. We were able to keep humor in the awkward moments, which made those moments a little lighter.

Becky Olson
Breast cancer survivor and national public speaker

Laughter really is a wonderful antidote. If you and your mate can keep your senses of humor especially when it comes to sex, you'll probably be able to talk about anything. However, you're going to have to take the cue from her because she might not be ready to laugh about it yet.

In the meantime, Becky Olson has developed a "honey do" list for husbands or partners of women with cancer. Perhaps some of her suggestions will be helpful (see www.breastfriends.com/about_us for a complete list).

1. *Give her Hugs and Kisses!*
2. Listen to her without judgment. Don't try to fix this; it can't be fixed.
3. Bring home her favorite takeout, light some candles, and enjoy each other.
4. Steal away in the middle of the day for a matinee or a lunch date.
5. Call her and tell her something funny. Remind her that you love her.
6. *Give her Kisses and Hugs!*
7. Write her a love note; tell her some future plans you want to share together.
8. Take her to hit a bucket of golf balls, or go for a drive in the country.
9. Touch her often and more than in a sexual way, she wants to know you still find her attractive and want to be with her.
10. And finally, keep telling her you love her and that you aren't going any-where. She might test your love at times, so make sure you communicate with words and deeds.

NOW, DO YOU HAVE A MINUTE TO TALK?

She is going to ask you this question soon. Now you know a little bit about why she wants to talk with you. Think about what you've wanted to tell her too. Remember that even if she is a strong woman, she probably needs to hear how much you still love her and are attracted to her since treatment. She needs to know if you want to resume an active sex life with her when she is ready. She needs to hear that you value her and that her concerns matter, even if she has misinterpreted your behavior or words.

If the two of you have not openly discussed sex in the past, it might be difficult to suddenly start this type of conversation. Most of us do not openly discuss our sex lives. To begin with, you can communicate through letters if this will help get the conversation started. It's important, however, that you eventually talk face-to-face about your sex life and what each of you wants and needs.

Your wife or partner is moving forward to good health and sexual vitality. She needs your help on this journey. When you are unsure how to help, try to think about how she would treat you if the roles were reversed. One thing cancer teaches us is that life is fleeting. As she makes her way to living her "new normal" life, try to give her the same love and understanding you know she would give to you if you were the one who had been sick. In relationships, as in marriage, none of us has all of the answers, and we can't always fix everything. What is important and what makes us stronger is taking the journey together.

❖

FACT OR FICTION?

"Sex will never be as good after cancer."

FICTION! Many couples enjoy a more intimate and fulfilling sex life after a life-threatening disease like cancer. Exploring new ways to find pleasure can actually enhance your sex life compared to the way it was before cancer.

---

[1] Silver M (2004). Breast Cancer Husband: How to Help Your Wife (And Yourself) Through Diagnosis, Treatment, and Beyond, pp. 272–293. New York: Rodale, Inc. Emmaus, PA: Rodale Press Incorporated.

Twelve

Hidden Blessings

Everything can be taken from a man or a woman but one thing: the last of human freedoms is to choose one's attitude in any given set of circumstances, to choose one's own way.[1]

Viktor Frankl

In <u>Man's Search for Meaning</u>

How could there possibly be any blessings in having had cancer? If blessings do exist, they've likely been hiding. Discovering each blessing is a true epiphany...that "Ah ha!" moment of clarity, when something valuable begins to emerge from the ashes.

For many women, cancer helps sharpen our focus on what we should be doing with our lives. We understand life is fragile and precious, so we begin to live a more purposeful life. After cancer, we may become acutely aware of each moment. Others may continue to live their lives in a blur of subconscious activity...but not us...at least we hope not. Cancer causes us to seize the day if we are wise. Sometimes some of us take a little longer to slow down, and realize what is important. If cancer teaches us anything, it teaches us what is important.

Our power lies in our ability to "choose our own way." When we decide to continue participating in life, and enjoy planning future events and living our lives to the fullest, we win. For instance, if you are reading this book, you are a champion. You've consciously chosen to continue living a full and meaningful life, even if you must work at it. You are undeniably resilient!

RESILIENCY, ANYONE?

All the wonders you seek are within yourself.
Sir Thomas Browne

Psychologists and others interested in the human condition have spent years studying "resiliency" in adults, adolescents, and in whole communities. Resiliency is defined as the "capacity for successful adaptation, positive functioning, or competence despite high risk, chronic stress, or following prolonged or severe trauma."[2] In other words, if you are able to adjust your thinking or way of doing things and adapt to your current situation, then you are resilient. Resiliency is about living your life as fully as possible in spite of being terrified, wounded, or broken.

What makes one person resilient in the face of trauma and another person fall to pieces? Is it sheer determination and will power or a strong sense of self? Not necessarily. And is there any real benefit to being resilient, other than tuning in to our innate survival instinct? The short answer is, "Yes!"

Resiliency is not about putting on a happy face when your spirit is broken. It's not about simply choosing to see the sunny side of life. As you are all too aware, cancer, its treatment, and its possible subsequent side effects can be devastating; you have every right to feel overwhelmed by them. You can cry, be angry and afraid, or even stay in bed if you feel like it…it's just that you can't remain there and be resilient at the same time.

Perhaps the key characteristic of resiliency is your ability to *adapt* to what is happening in your life, no matter how devastating. It's not necessarily about overcoming the damage done to your body, mind, and spirit, but it is about learning to cope with the changes. Adapting won't make it all go away…but it might make it easier for you to live with your circumstances. For instance, if you are unable to have sexual intercourse, finding pleasurable new ways to enjoy sex and making the necessary changes are examples of resiliency. It is about coping with and adapting to the challenges life hands you.

Spending long periods of time longing for "the good old days," or pining for who you once were, can be harmful. You have the power within you to decide whether to continue grieving for the past or to move forward by adapting to the way things are now. You could decide that you won't have any kind of sexual contact with your partner if it can't be the same as it once was. Or, you could knowingly decide that exploring new ways to enjoy one another sexually is an adventure you'd like to take together. We're not saying this choice is without its challenges, but we do know you can make the choice when you're ready.

> *Resiliency is not about putting on a happy face when your spirit is broken. It is about coping with and adapting to the challenges life hands you.*

For example, if breast stimulation was an important aspect of foreplay for you, but now your breasts are missing or numb, your partner may need to adapt by finding new erogenous zones. One of the hidden "blessings" of this kind of resilience is that you may discover brand new ways of making love that are even more satisfying than your old way. You wouldn't have known about these new pleasures otherwise.

Open communication may improve overall intimacy in your relationship. What is more intimate than discussing sexual pleasures with one another? Getting to know one another again, with or without sexual contact, can deepen your existing relationship and make you closer than you ever thought possible. Resiliency through adaptation can be a wonderful choice.

Robert Lifton is a psychiatrist who studied the resiliency of the survivors of Hiroshima and the Holocaust.[3] He found that resilient people commonly seek consistency in their lives after the traumatic event, remain connected to human events, and search for spiritual meaning in their lives. It doesn't mean that you won't ever get overwhelmed when stressful circumstances enter your life; it's just that you might have a better understanding of positive ways to cope with those events.

Other research indicates that, as a result of the cancer experience, resilience and growth may promote a sense of well-being. Even when a person is in poor health, she can be psychologically healthy and happy.[4] In fact, finding positive meaning in the cancer experience is widespread. Re-thinking your values and life's goals as a result of cancer may make you more satisfied with yourself and with your entire life.

Resilient people don't see themselves as victims. They refuse to hand over their beliefs and values, even during times of despair. They make an effort to find purpose and meaning in their lives, no matter what the circumstances. Asserting control over how you live your life, including your love life, may empower you to become resilient.

BLESSED STORIES

Some women find the strength to make big changes in their lives from their cancer experience. For example, they find the courage to leave an overly demanding job or a bad marriage. Some women begin doing the things on their list of "Things I Want to Do Before I Die" that they wrote when they were 20 years old. One woman we spoke to became an acrobatic pilot after cancer. Another swam with dolphins. It doesn't matter what your desire is, the important thing is to fulfill your dreams and life goals.

The changes you make, however, don't have to be big. If your life is fulfilling as it is, no changes may be necessary. Just living in the moment, appreciating those you love and those who love you, and understanding the blessings of your life may be all of the fulfillment that you need. The cancer experience may have shown you just how much you truly have already!

FLIGHT FOR LIFE

Sue Merrill, R.N., is an oncology case manager in Corvallis, Oregon. Sue explains that some women take time after cancer to review their marriages, and some discover they are not getting what they need from the husband they always thought of as supportive.

Sue tells us that several former patients left their husbands after cancer. She calls this act the "Flight for Life" phenomenon. Sue explains, "The whole person needs to be nurtured. Women go through cancer in a non-nurturing marriage and after treatment is completed, decide to leave the marriage." Sue talks to her patients about the importance of nurturing the whole person, and this includes their sex life. "A woman needs to feel loved and cherished and desirable. Look at the whole person when looking at yourself. You are not a disease. You are a loved and cherished woman."

In addition, Sue explains that it is common for women to have residual trauma after cancer. Your symptoms may not show up for years; suddenly you find yourself grieving your losses after being strong for everyone else around you. Others will think you ought to be better and get on with life, but you may actually get worse emotionally. People will say, "You're cured now," but as Sue explains, you may *not* be cured yet, at least not emotionally. You need to know this is normal for some women and that it's okay to grieve. Sue tells us, in her experience, a woman needs to work through it to get better. She also needs the support of her husband and family at that time, although it may be hard for them to understand why she is grieving her cancer so late. Many marriages can become troubled if the support is not there.

A NEW FOCUS

The cancer experience was a hidden blessing for Kathy LaTour because she learned her life's mission during the process. Cancer gave her a clear focus on what she was supposed to do next Not only did Kathy end up writing a passionate, caring book for women with breast cancer, she also developed a one-woman play called "One Mutant Cell," which is a humorous account of her cancer journey. Kathy's blessings came with her resilience and ability to make necessary but difficult choices after cancer.

Another successful example of finding the hidden blessings is Becky Olson, author and professional public speaker. Becky's career was the focus of big change after cancer. Becky was a successful major accounts advertising consultant. She made a great deal of income but was unable to spend much time with her family. Her position was very stressful, but like many people, Becky felt she was making too much money to leave. Then she developed cancer for the second time. Becky had been developing a different passion and finally got up the courage to resign her position. She eventually followed her passion into a new career and was able to focus full-time on what she loves...humorous public speaking! She now speaks to other women including those diagnosed with cancer about the changes in her own life and most importantly, about *hope*.

Becky survived two different battles with breast cancer. She learned the stress of her former job, as well as the medications for estrogen reduction, made her more fatigued and contributed to the loss of her sex drive. Becky still battles with the side-affects of her medication, but at least one thing has been resolved. Once she quit her job, Becky felt less tired, and her desire for intimacy also increased.   Without that second bout of cancer, Becky may have continued working at her former demanding job without fulfilling her life's passion.   And we wouldn't have the pleasure of her humorous presentations about having had cancer. We don't wish for the cancer, but Kathy and Becky are wonderful examples of finding its hidden blessings.

Cindy Smith was 43 years old and living in North Carolina when diagnosed with breast cancer. As it happened, Cindy's doctor was leading a study on treating the exact type and size of tumor that she had. Cindy was able to participate in a less invasive therapy as a result. During this time, Cindy began to reconsider her entire life and realized that she needed to make some changes. The first change Cindy made was to move across the country to Seattle.

Cindy quickly found new friends and surrounded herself with positive people leading very active lives. She said that one of the things she did was immediately tell new friends that she was a breast cancer patient. Talking about it helped her open up about her condition, not because she wanted the attention, but because as Cindy says, "The more you tell people about it, the more people open up. It seems people are afraid to talk about cancer. They must understand that it's just another disease that some people have to go through." By being open about her cancer, Cindy found support from new friends who appreciated her sharing this personal information.

Cindy's hidden blessings came when the cancer diagnosis forced her to reconsider the course of her life. She began asking, "What I am doing?" and "Why I am behaving like this?" as her own mortality lay in front of her. Even though the doctors had reassured her that she was not going to die, she could not help thinking that she might. Her diagnosis caused her to do the things she had always wanted to do but had not yet done. Cindy left North Carolina, bought a house in Seattle, and enrolled in Interior Design school, something she had always wanted to do.

Cindy suggests to other women going through cancer to try to realize that they will not have all of the answers right away. It takes time. At first, Cindy was not able to openly talk about her diagnosis and the subsequent changes. Cindy also found that validation as a woman came from within first, and then from others such as family and friends, and not only from men.

ADDITIONAL BLESSINGS...

Becky also tells us how her friends came to her rescue one day, and the blessings that came from it were surprising. Becky had lost all of her hair from chemotherapy and was having a difficult time with it. One day, her friend Patty surprised her with a gift from her husband Dennis. It was a hat with the words, "No Hair Day," plastered across the brim. It was on that day that Becky says she started laughing again. The end blessing was that Becky shares her story with other women in similar circumstances in her book, <u>The Hat That Saved My Life</u>.

Many women report a return to their faith, or experiencing a deepening of their faith, after cancer. Facing the possibility of death, no matter how remote, calls attention to this part of our lives. The blessings of a renewed or strengthened faith can blanket us in comfort and seep helpfully into every other area of our lives after cancer.

> ❖ *The blessings of a renewed or strengthened faith can blanket us in comfort and seep helpfully into every other area of our lives after cancer.*

Maybe one of the most common blessings from cancer is the clarity that often comes through the journey. It's when you realize that you are worthy and that you are so much more than a cancer diagnosis. You are a phenomenal woman, remember? You are valuable whatever your shape, size, color, religion, sexual orientation, or ethnicity. You have specific talents and abilities and a place in this world. Embrace all that you are; hopefully, the hidden blessings of cancer have at least taught you that this much is true.

Cancer may help you decide to live each day in the moment, appreciating who you are; you'll then get to experience another blessing from cancer called "post-traumatic" growth. As Viktor Frankl said in his book, <u>Man's Search for Meaning</u>, we can turn suffering into achievement and accomplishment. This is not the same as "being positive," or rising above the crisis when we're not yet ready. Post-traumatic growth is also not about subjecting ourselves to the "positive police" that we mentioned previously. No, it is so much more. Post-traumatic growth is about finding greater meaning in your life after cancer.

POST-TRAUMATIC GROWTH

All truths are easy to understand once they are discovered; the point is to discover them.

Galileo

It's true, positive changes *can* come from a cancer diagnosis and its sometimes grueling treatment. Eventually, you may respond to the unpleasant experience by moving to a higher level of functioning.

What is a "higher level of functioning?" It does *not* mean that you *ever* have to be *"happy"* that you had cancer. Moving to a higher level of functioning does mean, however, that you begin to see the benefits that come from having had cancer. You understand the lessons that cancer has taught you about your worth and value in this world.

Researchers have found that some patients experienced a greater meaning in and appreciation for life following cancer. In general, these studies suggested that after cancer, some people gain wisdom, personal growth, and positive personality changes, along with more meaningful and productive lives.[5 & 6]

What is interesting is that people can experience post-traumatic growth even while they are still going through trauma. Usually, these people have coped with the trauma by seeking guidance or by talking to others about their experience. It also helps to find meaning in your experience. This means that you should probably not keep your anxiety about having cancer to yourself; talk about it with someone you trust. Also, comments like, "look on the bright side," or, "keep a positive attitude," are not at all helpful. These messages may only tempt you to "stuff" your feelings even deeper, which won't help you in the long run.

Ask yourself, "What is my own personal growth since cancer?" What "hidden blessings" have you possibly overlooked? Spend some time writing down, or thinking about, aspects of your life that you think have changed for the better. Your marriage or partnership may have become more intimate simply due to better communication. You may learn to look out for your own needs while you are looking out for those you love. You may decide to start checking off items on your list of things you wanted to do in your life. You may simply learn to live for today and let tomorrow take care of itself. But really, this is a list for you to write for yourself. You may be surprised by what you see there. It's really worth taking the time to do this.

AND THEY'RE OFF...TO THE RACES?

Cancer helps some women take charge of their lives. You may participate in a new, symbolic activity that empowers you after cancer. A great example of this is amateur Dragon Boat racing.

Dragon Boat racing began in China over 2,000 years ago. People raced in narrow, long boats in hopes of encouraging rain to fall for the harvest and to avoid hardship. The Asian dragon is a symbol of water, and it is believed to rule the sea and control the rain. Over time, another story emerged about the Dragon Boat.

Legend has it that a famous Chinese poet, Qu Yaun, was banished from his country by the King. He spent many years writing poetry until one day, his heart broken, he clung to a large rock and threw himself into the river. Because he was beloved by his countrymen, they all jumped into their boats in a race to save him, banging on drums and splashing their paddles to keep the fish away from his body. Today, Dragon Boat races are celebrations that include drums, splashing paddles, and colorful boats.

Many women who've had cancer join a Dragon Boat team to empower themselves and celebrate their lives after cancer. The boats are full of women who have survived cancer. In the United States, one of the oldest Dragon Boat clubs made up of cancer survivors is the Wasabi Paddling Club (www.wasabiusa.org); many other Dragon Boat teams exist throughout the U.S. and Canada. Many Canadian women who have survived cancer have been quite active in Dragon Boat racing for years. An example of a Canadian Dragon Boat racing team is the Canadians Abreast, located at: www.canadiansabreast.abcn.ca. To find a Dragon Boat team in your area or to learn more about it, visit the Web site: en.wikipedia.org/wiki/Dragon_boat_racing.

Dragon Boat teams spread awareness of women's cancers, often breast cancer, and encourage survivors to grab hold of their lives with gusto. Many women report not only physical, but also mental and spiritual benefits from being part of a Dragon Boat team. Even if you don't chose to join a Dragon Boat team, doing something right now that you've always wanted to do may lift your spirits and release the wild side of you!

AT LAST...THE GRAND FINALE!

Losing one horse might gain you a better horse.

Chinese proverb

What better "horse" do you need in your life? Is it an external "horse," like the job you always wanted or a way out of a bad relationship? Maybe it's an internal "horse," such as having the courage to ask for what you want or to accept and love yourself just as you are. Either way, life after cancer is different...hopefully, better. We hope after reading this book that your love life significantly improves, both physically and emotionally. We hope you get everything your heart desires, and that you do what you have to do to make that happen.

Whether we like it or not, cancer has a profound influence on our lives. It molds us into new people. You've been given the opportunity to see everything differently, perhaps even more clearly than others who have not experienced what you have been through. You can let it break you, or you can choose to rise to the occasion when you are ready. Everything about your life can be new or renewed. Again, it's not about the "positive police" or being a cheerleader. It's about evaluating your life, understanding what you want from it, and going after it when you have the energy and desire to achieve your goals.

I wouldn't wish cancer on my worst enemy. Yet, my life is fuller from the experience. When I finally began to see the blessings that have come into my life since cancer, I was over-whelmed with gratefulness...not for the cancer, but for all it has taught me.

Laura*, 62

Hey, I learned that reconstructed breasts don't bounce when I am jogging or doing aerobics! I hardly need the expensive sports bras I once had to buy.

Brooke*, 39

I learned I was married to the best man on the planet. My daughter had dyed my hair orange because we knew it would fall out soon, and we were having a little fun with it first. Later, I was in the shower when all of my hair fell out except two tufts on either side of my ears. I stood there, in the shower, crying. I was quite a sight: one tight, rubbery breast from radiation, and the other controlled by gravity. I wasn't overweight, just under height, with a long chemo tube dangling from my breast to my waist. I was bald, with two tufts of orange hair sticking out from around my ears.

My husband flew up the stairs, saw me in all my glory, then quickly wrapped me in a towel and told me to go downstairs and wait for him. He cleaned up all of the hair from the shower, came downstairs with clippers, and shaved the two ridiculous tufts of orange hair off my head. Then, without warning, he turned the razor onto his own head and shaved his head bald too.

Becky Olson

We encourage you to find the blessings and the humor where you can in your current situation, especially in your love life. After talking with your doctor, remember to bring lubricants, towels, a vibrator, good communication skills, and especially your sense of humor as you and your partner write your new sexual script.

Remember what you've read here. May you safely find your way back to a satisfying love life, and may the journey include all the blessings you are looking for!

Character cannot be developed in ease and quiet. Only through experience of trial and suffering can the soul be strengthened, ambition inspired, and success achieved.

Helen Keller
(Reprinted Courtesy American Foundation for the Blind)

[1] Frankl V (2000). <u>Man's Search for Meaning</u>. Boston: Beacon Press.

[2] Egeland B, Carlson E, et al. (1993). Resilience As Process. <u>Development and Psychopathology</u>, 5(4): 517.

[3] Lifton RJ (1993). <u>The Protean Self: Human Resilience In An Age Of Fragmentation.</u> Chicago: University of Chicago Press.

[4] Wenzel LB, Donnelly JP, et al. (2002). Resilience, Reflection, And Residual Stress In Ovarian Cancer Survivorship: A Gynecologic Oncology Group Study. <u>Psychooncology</u>, 11(2): 142-153.

[5] Cordova MJ, Andrykowski MA (2004). Responses To Cancer Diagnosis And Treatment: Posttraumatic Stress And Posttraumatic Growth. <u>Seminars in Clinical Neuropsychology</u>, 8(4): 286-296.

[6] Ho SM, Chan CL, Ho RT (2004). Posttraumatic Growth In Chinese Cancer Survivors. <u>Psychooncology</u>, 13(6): 377-389.

RESOURCE LIST

We have compiled a few available resources that may help. The list is not a complete list, and you may find other resources that are more helpful than those mentioned here. These resources are listed in alphabetical order, and we do not recommend one over another.

The information provided was current as of publication, but it is subject to change. Don't despair if you can't reach a particular organization. There are many helping hands waiting for your call. In fact, there are more organizations and discussion groups than the ones listed here, so please reach out until you find the one that fits you best.

BOOKS

For You:

Affirmations, Meditations & Encouragements for Women Living With Breast Cancer, by Linda Dackman.

After Breast Cancer: A Common-Sense Guide to Life After Treatment, by Hester Hill Schnipper, LICSW

The Breast Cancer Companion: From Diagnosis To Recovery: Everything You Need to Know Along the Way, by Kathy LaTour.

Can't Buy Me Love: How Advertising Changes the Way We Think and Feel, by Jean Kilbourne

Couples Confronting Cancer: Keeping Your Relationship Strong, by Joy L. Fincannon, R.N., M.S. and Katherine V. Bruss, Psy.D.

The Hat That Saved My Life, by Becky Olson

Living Beyond Breast Cancer: A Survivor's Guide for When Treatment Ends and the Rest of Your Life Begins, by Marisa Weiss, M.D., and Ellen Weiss

Let Me Count the Ways, by Marty Klein, Ph.D. and Riki Robbins, Ph.D.

Love Your Looks, by Carolynn Hillman

Passionate Marriage, David Schnarch

Sexuality and Fertility After Cancer, by Leslie R. Schover, Ph.D.

Sexuality and Cancer: For the Woman Who Has Cancer and Her Partner, by the American Cancer Society (free brochure).

The Sexy Years: Discover the Hormone Connection: The Secret to Fabulous Sex, Great Health, and Vitality, For Women and Men, by Suzanne Summers

Up Front: Sex and the Post-Mastectomy Woman, by Linda Dackman (this book is out of print but well worth finding it at your local library or from a used book seller)

Uplift: Secrets from the Sister of Breast Cancer Survivors, by Barbara Delinsky

What Doctors Didn't Tell Us: About Double Breasted Suits and Single Breasted Women, by Martha Falterman, Loretta Schultz, and Neppie Trahan

Why Men Don't Listen, and Women Can't Read Maps, by Allan and Barbara Pease

Women and Cancer Magazine, subscribe at: patient.cancerconsultants.com/wac/

For Your Male Partner:

Breast Cancer Husband: How to Help Your Wife (and Yourself) Through Diagnosis, Treatment, and Beyond, by Marc Silver.

Man to Man: When the Woman You Love Has Breast Cancer, by Andy Murcia (husband of actress Anne Jillian) and Bob Stewart.

For Your Loved Ones and Friends:

The Etiquette of Illness, by Susan P. Halpern

Cancer Etiquette: What to Say and Do When Someone You Know or Love Has Cancer, by Rosanne Kalick.

LINGERIE, LUBRICANTS, VIBRATORS, AND MORE

The following are lingerie and specialty shops that sell products online for women with special needs after cancer treatment, such as lingerie with pockets to insert a drainage tube, ostomy bag, or to cover a missing breast. Additionally, some of the stores identified sell vibrators and vaginal dilators, although be sure to check with your doctor before trying these products. You may prefer other stores in your local area, or other online stores than those mentioned here.

Babeland at www.babeland.com

Eve's Garden at www.evesgarden.com

Good Vibes at www.goodvibes.com

Just Like a Woman at www.justlikeawoman.com

Make Me Heal at www.makemeheal.com

My Pleasure at www.mypleasure.com

Notti Wear at www.nottiwear.com

TrueLife, which *also* sells breast forms, at www.camphealthcare.com

Ultimate Moments at www.intimatemomentsapparel.com

Vaginismus Products at www.vaginismus.com/products/dilator_set/

Various sexual aid products at www.walgreens.com

WHI Lubricating Gel, by calling 1-800-537-8658

Wound, Ostomy & Continence Nurses Society (WOCN) at www.wocn.org/patients/specialty_items.html

Xandria Collection at www.xandria.com

Zestra at www.zestraforwomen.com

Helpful Web Sites

The following Web sites may be great resources to obtain other helpful information. Again, this list is not a complete list of what is available, and we do not recommend one above another.

Breast Cancer support information at www.breastcancer.org

Breast Friends at www.breastfriends.com, which offers support advice for best friends and partners.

Becky Olson, cancer survivor and humorist speaker, at www.beckyolson.com

Canadian Breast Cancer Network (CBCN) at www.cbcn.ca or 1-800-685-8820 (in Canada).

Canadian Cancer Society at www.cancer.ca or (416) 961-7223

Canadian Breast Cancer Foundation at www.cbcf.org or (416) 596-6773 or toll-free 1 (800) 387-9816

CancerConsultants at www.cancerconsultants.com, which provides current cancer health information for patients and oncology professionals.

Dragon Boat Racing Teams information: Go to www.boatowners.com/canoe_dragonboats.htm to find information about a dragon boat team in your area.

EduCare Web site at website: www.cancerhelp.com, which offers general education about women's cancers and their treatments.

Eyes on the Prize at www.eyesontheprize.org/index.shtml, which offers general support and information about gynecological cancers.

Look Good...Feel Better at www.lookgoodfeelbetter.org, which is an organization that provides "makeovers" for cancer survivors to help with body image and self-esteem.

National Cancer Institute at www.cancer.gov, which provides general information on cancer and its treatment.

Network for Excellence in Women's Sexual Health at www.newshe.com, which provides general information on women's sexual health by Drs. Laura and Jennifer Berman.

Reach to Recovery program, American Cancer Society at www. cancer.org/docroot/ESN/content/ESN_3_1x_Reach_to_Recovery_5.asp?sitearea=ESN, which is run by cancer survivor volunteers and helps improve body image, self-esteem, and resources for breast prostheses.

Sloan-Kettering Sexual Health program: www.mskcc.org/mskcc/html/13814.cfm (or check your local cancer center for information).

UCLA Sexual Medicine Center (310) 794-3030, which provides information about developing treatments for female sexual dysfunction.

Women to Women at www.womentowomen.com, which provides general information on women's health.

Web site For Men:

Men Against Breast Cancer at www.menagainstbreastcancer.org

General Cancer Information And Support

National Cancer Institute
www.cancer.gov, 800-4-CANCER (800-422-6237)

American Cancer Society (ACS)
800-ACS-2345 (800-227-2345), www.cancer.org

American Society of Clinical Oncology (ASCO)
703-299-0150, www.asco.org

Asian and Pacific Islander Cancer Education Materials (APICEM)
800-ACS-2345 (800-227-2345), www.cancer.org/apicem

Association of Cancer Online Resources
(212)-226-5525, www.acor.org

Bloch Cancer Hotline
800-433-0464, www.blochcancer.org

Canadian Breast Cancer Foundation
www.cbcf.org, (416) 596-6773 or toll-free 1 (800) 387-9816

Canadian Breast Cancer Network
www.cbcn.ca, 800-685-8820

Canadian Cancer Society
(416) 961-7223, www.cancer.ca

Cancer411.org (clinical trials information)
877-226-2741, www.cancer411.org

CancerCare, Inc.
800-813-HOPE (800-813-4673), www.cancercare.org

CancerConsultants.com
www.cancerconsultants.com

Cancer Hope Network
877-HOPENET (877-467-3638), www.cancerhopenetwork.org

CancerSource
www.cancersource.com

ChemoCare.com
www.chemocare.com

Corporate Angel Network, Inc.
866-328-1313, www.corpangelnetwork.org

Fertile Hope
888-994-4673 , www.fertilehope.org

Gilda's Club, Inc.
888-GILDA-4U (888-445-3248), www.gildasclub.org

Mautner Project (women who partner with women)
866-MAUTNER (866-628-8637), www.mautnerproject.org

National Comprehensive Cancer Network (NCCN)
215-690-0300, www.nccn.org

OncoLink
www.oncolink.com

People Living With Cancer
703-797-1914, www.plwc.org

Planet Cancer
www.planetcancer.org

Team Survivor
www.teamsurvivor.org

Ulman Cancer Fund for Young Adults
888-393-FUND (3863), www.ulmanfund.org

Vital Options and "The Group Room" Cancer Radio Talk Show
800-GRP-ROOM (800-477-7666), www.vitaloptions.org

The Wellness Community
888-793-WELL (888-793-9355), www.thewellnesscommunity.org

Women's Cancer Network (WCN)
312-578-1439, www.wcn.org

COMPLEMENTARY THERAPIES

About Herbs, Botanicals & Other Products
www.mskcc.org/mskcc/html/11570.cfm

National Center for Complementary and Alternative Medicine
(NCCAM)
888-644-6226, www.nccam.nih.gov

Smith Farm Center for Healing and the Arts
202-483-8600, www.SmithFarm.com

American Pain Foundation
888-615-7246, www.painfoundation.org

ADVOCACY ORGANIZATIONS

LIVESTRONG
512-236-8820, www.livestrong.org

National Coalition for Cancer Survivorship
877-622-7937, www.canceradvocacy.org

Patient Advocate Foundation (PAF)
800-532-5274, www.patientadvocate.org

Breast, Ovarian and Gynecologic Cancers

Breastcancer.org
www.breastcancer.org

US Department of Health and Human Services, Breast Cancer Information
877-696-6775, www.hhs.gov/breastcancer

HER2Support.org (HER2-Positive Breast Cancer)
760-602-9178, www.her2support.org

JACOB International (Jews Against Cancer of the Breast)
561-394-9100, www.jacobintl.org

Living Beyond Breast Cancer
610-645-4567, www.lbbc.org

Sharsheret (young Jewish women with breast cancer)
866-474-2774, www.sharsheret.org

Sisters Network, Inc.
866-781-1808, www.sistersnetworkinc.org/index.htm

Susan G. Komen Breast Cancer Foundation
800-I'M AWARE (800-462-9273), www.komen.org

Y-ME National Breast Cancer Organization, Inc.
800-221-2141 (English), 800-986-9505 (Spanish), www.y-me.org

Young Survival Coalition
877-972-1011, www.youngsurvival.org

National Ovarian Cancer Coalition (NOCC)
888-OVARIAN (888-682-7426), www.ovarian.org

Gynecologic Cancer Foundation
(312) 578-1439, www.thegcf.org

MYELOMA, LEUKEMIA AND LYMPHOMA, AND MYELODYSPLASTIC SYNDROMES

Aplastic Anemia & MDS International Foundation, Inc.
800-747-2820, www.aamds.org

Cutaneous Lymphoma Foundation
248-644-9014, www.clfoundation.org

International Myeloma Foundation
800-452-CURE (800-452-2873), www.myeloma.org

The Leukemia and Lymphoma Society
800-955-4572, www.lls.org

Lymphoma Research Foundation (LRF)
800-500-9976 , www.lymphoma.org

Multiple Myeloma Research Foundation (MMRF)
203-972-1250, www.multiplemyeloma.org

OTHER CANCERS

Bladder Cancer Advocacy Network
301-469-6865, www.bcan.org

American Brain Tumor Association
800-886-2282 , www.abta.org

The Brain Tumor Foundation
800-934-CURE (2873), www.braintumorfoundation.org

The Brain Tumor Society
800-770 8287 , www.tbts.org

᠁nal Brain Tumor Foundation (NBTF)
CURE (800-934-2873), www.braintumor.org

Caring for Carcinoid Foundation
www.caringforcarcinoid.org, (857) 222-5492

C3: Colorectal Cancer Coalition
202-244-2906, www.c-three.org

Colon Cancer Alliance
877-422-2030, www.ccalliance.org

Lung Cancer Alliance
800-298-2436 , www.lungcanceralliance.org

Melanoma International Foundation
888-463-6663, www.melanomaintl.org

The Melanoma Research Foundation (MRF)
800-MRF-1290, www.melanoma.org

The Skin Cancer Foundation
800-754-6490 , www.skincancer.org

It's Time to Focus on Lung Cancer
877-646-5864, www.lungcancer.org

Liddy Shriver Sarcoma Initiative
www.liddyshriversarcomainitiative.org

The Sarcoma Alliance
415-381-7236, www.sarcomaalliance.com

ThyCa: Thyroid Cancer Survivors' Association
877-588-7904, www.thyca.org

FOR MEN: PROSTATE CANCER SUPPORT ORGANIZATIONS

American Foundation for Urologic Disease (AFUD)
800-242-2383, www.afud.org

Prostate Cancer Foundation
1-800-757-CURE (2873), www.prostatecancerfoundation.org

The Prostate Net
888-4-776-7638, www.prostate-online.com

US TOO! International, Inc.
800-80-US TOO (800-808-7866), www.ustoo.org